THE COMPLETE
GUIDE TO

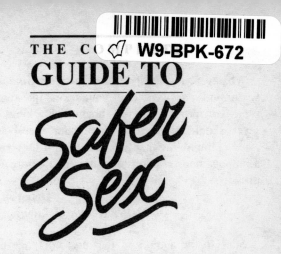

Safer Sex

The most strikingly honest, ethical, practical, authoritative primer on sex available ever! There is nothing else as complete and *useable* in this time of increased fear of sexual disease. This publication does more than just deal with disease, however, it addresses sexual health in a real way.

Quite frankly, this is the book we have all wanted but many probably will be afraid to so admit.

For your own health and life, for your clients' health and life, for your family's health and life, for society's health and life, do yourself and all of us a favor—read it soon!

This guide need only one thing—that is, immediate wide-spread dissemination.

Richard L. Bennett, M.D., Ph.D.
FACOG, Akron, OH

Whatever your lifestyle, the *Complete Guide to Safer Sex* provides answers to all your sexual questions—plus some you probably never thought of asking! Chapter seven should be required reading for everybody interested in improving their sex life, even if they've been in a monogamous relationship since long before AIDS hit the scene.

Deborah Quilter
Better Health & Living **magazine**

Stars to the authors of the most complete *Complete Guide to Safer Sex* I have ever seen. The book is so thorough that, for me as a professional, it will provide guidelines for answering countless questions.

It should be next to the KY jelly on everyone's bedstand.

Marilyn Volker, Ed.D.
Director,
Institute on Sexism and Sexuality
Miami, FL

This is an authoritative, competent review of current available information on AIDS, with advice and recommendations about human sexual interactions offered in a sensitive and positive manner. It conveys strong sex-positive messages and suggests many avenues for sexual expression that minimize or totally eliminate disease transmission risks. It is a book to own and to read and reread.

David McWhirter, M.D.
Former President,
Society for Scientific Study of Sex
San Diego, CA

An outstanding book. There is nothing quite like it on the market. It is very clearly written, relevant to the problems faced today by many different groups of people, and accurate in its reporting of research on AIDS.

It is imaginative in its suggestions regarding safe forms of sexuality and in presenting concrete ways of achieving a wider range of safe sexual outlets. If people want to learn about AIDS and how to protect themselves and want to read only one book—this is the one best source.

Ira L. Reiss, Ph.D.
Professor of Sociology, University of Minnesota,
Minneapolis

What I find most persuasive about this book is its deeply informed and dedicated effort, amidst the hysteria occasioned by the AIDS epidemic, to preserve the individual's freedom to manage her or his own sexuality. "Safe" and "safer" sex is not presented as medical prescription or unconditional warranty but as a specific decision point we face in future sexual encounters regardless of the number, social "identity," or "lifestyle" of our partners.

John P. De Cecco, Ph.D.
Professor of Psychology and
Human Sexuality Studies
Director, Center for Research
and Education in Sexuality,
San Francisco State University.

THE COMPLETE
GUIDE TO
Safer Sex

TED McILVENNA, M.Div., Ph.D.
Editor

Authored By Senior Faculty of The Institute
For Advanced Study of Human Sexuality:

Clark Taylor, Ph.D., Ed.D.
Research Director

Published by Barricade Books Inc.
Fort Lee, New Jersey

Published by Barricade Books Inc.
1530 Palisade Avenue
Fort Lee, NJ 07024

Distributed to the trade by Publishers Group West

ISBN 0-942637-58-5

Printed in the United States of America

Dedication

To all those who have fought and lost, and those who continue to fight the battle against AIDS and ARC. We are especially mindful of the sacrifices of those who have faced physical illness, emotional devastation, and political vengeance. The tragedy of all this is that it is taking place in a society that could mobilize resources but refuses to do so because of the misguided vested interests of antisexual forces.

THE COMPLETE
GUIDE TO
Safer Sex

Foreword

AIDS has become a test case for sexologists. Does their science have any practical application? Can it be put to any general use? Can it benefit society? If it cannot contribute to the fight against a sexually transmissible disease what good is it? Do we have to rely exclusively on medical research to protect us and to give us back our sexual options?

Fortunately, the answer to the last question is: NO! Sexology has been studying human sexual behavior for a very long time. As a science in its own right, it was established early in our century, and today it flourishes in many countries all over the world. This has become evident through the many international sexological congresses before World War II and through the World Congresses of Sexology since then, which have been held in Europe, the U.S., Israel, Asia and Latin America. It is now time for sexologists in all affected countries to speak up, to offer their particular expertise, and to get involved in AIDS prevention. At the same time, they should also inform and support each other through increased international cooperation.

Our Institute in San Francisco has been researching sexual behavior for many years, and we have, from the very beginning, sought out and kept close contact with people of all sexual lifestyles in all their different environments. We therefore know how wide the sexual spectrum is and how unique every individual.

We believe that, with proper concern and understanding, very many people who are now at risk for AIDS can be helped to change their sexual behavior and to avoid the risk of infection. What's more important: they can learn to do so to their own satisfaction!

This is the only approach that promises any hope in the long run, as long as no vaccine and no successful therapy are available.

We therefore hope that this book will be read as widely as possible and that all sexologists everywhere will unite in serving life by putting all of their efforts into preserving it.

Wardell B. Pomeroy, Ph.D.
Erwin J. Haeberle, Ph.D., Ed.D.

Editor's Foreword

A sexologist sees the world from a special perspective that makes the various sexual denial games people play seem sadly ridiculous. A sexologist assumes that everyone either has done or is capable of doing almost everything or anything. We look, we catalogue, and we are usually uninvolved experts. The AIDS crisis suddenly has pushed sexologists into the role of involved experts. We must, by necessity, become advocates for safe sex.

This is a moment in history when we are called to act. We are asking all other persons who are involved in servicing and influencing other humans to also become advocates of safe sex. For all of us who are captives in this hold of streets and years there is no hiding place down here.

For those involved in the delivery of sexual health services: You must make yourself an expert on safe sex.

For high schools, colleges and universities: You must offer classroom courses for credit on safe sex. You must provide resource materials including safe sex products in all of your student health services.

For churches: You must provide training for all clergy. In addition, develop education programs and resource centers with safe sex products.

For social service agencies: You must train your personnel and provide resource materials and safe sex products.

For City, County and State public health agencies: You must have trained personnel and education programs and safe sex products.

For the media: You must give up the snicker-and-giggle way you deal with sex and focus on the truth about the need for safe sex.

For law enforcement personnel: You must have training and information about where people can get information about safe sex and make informed referrals.

For the Justice Department: You must put aside your mission of search and destroy against the sex industry.

For the sex industry: You must sacrifice some of your profit and provide safe sex products at affordable prices.

For the entertainment industry: You must offer your considerable talents to the creations of the best and most entertaining educational programs on safe sex.

For the voluntary and involuntary funding services: You must seek out and help fund schools, clinics, etc. that advocate and field safe sex programs.

For businesses: You must provide education, resources and safe sex products for your workers and the time they need to learn about safe sex.

The military: You must provide comprehensive education, resources and safe sex products to our service people wherever they are in the world.

For the average person: You must allocate time and money to learn about and provide for safe sex products.

Dr. Wardell Pomeroy, the Academic Dean of our

Institute, more than any other person in the field of sexology has insisted that we operate from a stance of maximum sexual information. He tells a story of a beginning student who said he wanted to be a sexologist but there were certain things about sex that he didn't want to study. Dr. Pomeroy's reply was, "If that's the case, why did you come here?"

If you really don't want to learn about safe sex, this is the time to put this book aside. If you do want to learn about safe sex, then you have come to the right place.

Introduction

When The Institute for Advanced Study of Human Sexuality was asked to create a guide to safe sex, Institute President Ted McIlvenna was given the responsibility of putting together an "AIDS Task Force" of sexologists. Their task was to respond from a sex-positive perspective to an international health crisis. As the special AIDS panel of the National Academy of Sciences put it, "Sex education is no longer advice about reproductive choice, but has become advice about a life-or-death matter." They further said that if such a campaign of sex education was not launched by 1991, the Untied States would face a national health catastrophe with 50,000 Americans a year dying of AIDS. The World Health Organization also issued a report saying we could soon be facing 2 million deaths a year worldwide.

The former U.S. Surgeon General C. Everett Koop, and his successors, have called for a nationwide program to educate school children about AIDS, including candid information about how it is spread and how it can be avoided.

Dr. McIlvenna's criteria for the task force members were:

1) They had to be trained, professional sexologists with at least 10 years of fulltime work in the field of sexology.

2) They had to be academically qualified about sexual functioning, and in addition possess specialized knowledge about AIDS and other sexually transmitted diseases.

3) They had to have a special area of sexological expertise that could add to and benefit the whole-team approach.

Six persons were chosen, two women and four men. Modern movies have told us the story of super groups of people who are brought together to get a job done. These groups have been variously known as the Dirty Dozen, the Magnificent 7, A-Team, etc., so all of us understand a team approach to getting a job done. Following are some descriptions of our "Six for Safe Sex" Task Force.

Loretta Haroian, Ph.D. The world's leading expert on childhood and adolescent sexuality, Loretta was chosen for her genius in understanding how children and adolescents learn about sex and her ability to design learning methods that truly help these target groups.

David Lourea, Ed.D. David is on the team as a result of his years of experience in the design and direction of safe sex seminars and his ability to create the various games and exercises which can help people to develop safe sex practices.

Ted McIlvenna, M.Div., Ph.D. The administrator and convener of the Task Force, Ted is a theologian and sexologist committed to the integration of sexology with other academic disciplines.

Charles Moser, Ph.D., M.D. An expert on lifestyles and special sexual populations, Charlie brings to the team a reminder that our educational endeavor must be directed toward that huge range of lifestyles.

Maggi Rubenstein, Ph.D. Maggi has taught more people about sexuality in workshops than any other living person. Her special expertise is the integration of safe sex concerns and issues into the mainstream of sex education.

Clark Taylor, Ph.D., Ed.D. Often referred to as "Dr. Safe Sex," Clark has managed to acquire and make usable a vast anthology of interdisciplinary information about AIDS and other sexually transmitted diseases and the multitudes of attitudes and programs that have been designed and are in use throughout the world.

The first dilemma faced by the Task Force in the creation of *The Complete Guide to Safer Sex* was that age-old specter which haunts all sex education: How candid can we be about sexual matters? We have decided not to treat sex as a delicate subject. The Task Force has chosen a sexual ethic based on the science of human duty in its widest extent, including full disclosure on all matters dealing with the quality of life that maximizes freedom of choice.

The objectives of the Task Force are as follows:

1. First and foremost to keep people alive.
2. To present a digest of the latest available informa-

tion to enable you to determine your level of personal risk.

3. To provide as much sex-positive information as possible about AIDS and the ways of preventing its spread.

4. To provide safe sex techniques which as far as possible do not detract from the pleasure and meaning of sexuality.

5. To acknowledge and address different sexual life-styles and provide accurate information on how to use safe sex techniques that are particularly applicable to those lifestyles.

6. To provide programmed learning techniques and motivation to help you change from unsafe to safe sex techniques.

7. To empower you to explore and make informed decisions about your sexual lifestyle.

8. To provide practical and concrete alternatives and suggestions.

9. Finally, to provide an approach to AIDS that is in accord with basic human sexual rights.

Basic human rights must always be built around freedom of choice, for there can be no freedom if there is no choice. We are now at a special point in history where we can no longer indulge ourselves with antisexual moralistic baggage of the past which is no longer functional.

No matter which way we look at the health crisis caused by AIDS we come to the conclusion that we must move fast. Sexologists and other scientists agree that our Number One weapon is education. Sexual ignorance can no longer be seen as the equivalent of sexual innocence. Sexual ignorance is just plain ignorance.

A lot has been said about human rights, but little has been said about sexual rights. As sex education begins to takes its proper role in helping us all understand the human condition, the educational constructs must include basic sexual rights.

These Basic Sexual Rights, approved by the Ethics Committee of the Fifth World Congress of Sexology, are:

1. The freedom of any sexual thought, fantasy or desire.
2. The right to sexual entertainment, freely available in the marketplace, including sexually explicit materials dealing with the full range of sexual behavior.
3. The right not to be exposed to sexual material or behavior.
4. The right to sexual self-determination.
5. The right to seek out and engage in consensual sexual activity.
6. The right to engage in sexual acts or activities of any kind whatsoever, providing they do not involve nonconsensual acts, violence, constraint, coercion or fraud.
7. The right to be free of persecution, condemnation, discrimination, or societal intervention in private sexual behavior.

8. The recognition by society that every person, partnered or unpartnered, has the right to the pursuit of a satisfying consensual sociosexual life free from political, legal or religious interference and that there need to be mechanisms in society where the opportunities of sociosexual activities are available to the following: disabled persons; chronically ill persons; those incarcerated in prisons, hospitals or institutions; those disadvantaged because of age, lack of physical attractiveness, or lack of social skills; the poor and the lonely.

9. The basic right of all persons who are sexually dysfunctional to have available nonjudgemental sexual health care.

10. The right to control conception.

There are many voices calling for every type of extreme sexual repression. There are political forces that wish to control people by controlling their sexuality. There are religious voices that claim that AIDS is God's judgement against an immoral world. There are fanatics claiming that AIDS is history's final Armageddon. It seems that many people have charts for our sexuality. There is an old story about a young explorer who decided to go out and learn about the world. He found an old chart that had written all over it: Devils Be Here . . . Sinners Be Here . . . Heathens Be Here . . . Lepers Be Here. That young explorer took his pen and wrote in bold letters across the entire map: **The Spirit of Truth Be Here.** We are confident that AIDS can be prevented without violating the basic human sexual rights.

The authors of this book invite you to look carefully at the charts we have prepared and be guided by your own quest for truth as you evaluate and seek to find pleasure and meaning in your own sexuality, the sexuality of others and sexuality in our culture in the Age of AIDS.

ACKNOWLEDGMENTS

The Editor and writers acknowledge the support of The Institute faculty as a whole and specifically the counsel of Drs. Wardell B. Pomeroy and Erwin J. Haeberle.

In particular, we wish to acknowledge several people who have helped and encouraged us to develop a sexologist's approach to AIDS risk reduction. Margo Rila, Ed.D., a sexologist with the Women's AIDS Network, was particularly helpful in developing a women's perspective. Sam Puckett, Jackson Peyton, Les Pappas, David May and Chuck Frutchi of the San Francisco AIDS Foundation deserve special recognition for support over the years. We acknowledge and extend special thanks to Joani Blank for her inspiration in the workbook section of the text. And we wish to recognize Myrna Alma, Cynthia Slater and Mark Chester for their insightful help on the S/M portions of the book. Jim Garner deserves special recognition for his help measuring and testing condoms.

Of course there could be no book without Jean Amos, who facilitated preparation of the manuscript in all stages. Also assisting in this task of keeping us dedicated to logical sentence construction, was Ms. Melissa Haroian. We are particularly grateful to Buzz Bense for his artistic consultation, design and layout of the Guide, also for his patience.

In addition, we acknowledge the many lecturers, health officials, researchers and graduate students who have helped us understand the need to find workable ways to manage our sexuality in the Age of AIDS.

WARNING:

The language of polite society and the sexual language of the bedroom are often quite different. For reasons of effectiveness and clarity, we have decided to use both. While scientists may find long terms in foreign or dead languages thrilling, ordinary people often find this language a turnoff. A major purpose of the Guide is to help people turn on to safe sex. Thus when we are presenting material on creating an exciting safer sex lifestyle, we will sometimes use terms familiar to sexually active people, but seldom found in the tomes of academia. When we are presenting the more formal academic material, we will use the more traditional language of scholars. To help professionals become familiar and comfortable with the common sexual language and the layperson to better understand technical terms, a glossary has been included.

CHAPTER 1
Thinking About Sex and AIDS:
THE BASICS

What is AIDS—Are You At Risk?

The news has reported that AIDS is a health crisis, an epidemic and a plague. Media coverage has created virtual hysteria by speculating a geometric progression of AIDS will hypothetically kill everyone on earth at a given moment in the next century.

In fact, AIDS is at this time known to be caused by a virus that:

- Can be transmitted between people who share body fluids.
- Destroys the immune system.
- Is often fatal after it enters a person's body.
- Is easily killed before it enters the body.

The fear about AIDS centers around sexual activity because sex is the most common way of exchanging body fluids and because it was first identified as a disease among men engaging in homosexual activity. It is also used as an example of the divine consequences of sexual excesses by antisexual politicians and religionists.

The Complete Guide to Safer Sex is designed to help you understand what AIDS is and what it is not; to allow you to calculate your own personal level of risk; and to determine what changes, if any, you may need to make in your sexual pattern or lifestyle to give you peace of mind.

Sexual activity, including exchange of body fluids, is **not dangerous** if neither you nor your partner carries the AIDS virus. That fact is reassuring. However, determining whether or not a person has or has not been exposed to the virus may create quite a problem.

People's sexuality is one of the most private aspects of their lives. Most people are reluctant, if not unwilling, to reveal their innermost sexual secrets. They may be embarrassed, ashamed, or feel that full disclosure might hurt their partner, restrict their freedom, or jeopardize their chances of a sexual encounter.

- Men who relate to other men often have difficulty communicating about their personal health concerns and past unsafe sexual activity.
- Many men have in the past or continue on occasion to have sex with prostitutes even though they are in a committed relationship or married. Prostitutes are at high risk for AIDS.
- Many married men and women have casual sex or ongoing sexual affairs with partners who are having sex with others who may be in high risk groups.
- Many heterosexual women and men have occasional or periodic sexual encounters with homosexual or

bisexual men. Gay and bisexual men are at high risk for AIDS.

- A new sexual partner may be or may have been a needle sharing intravenous drug user. People who share needles are at high risk for AIDS.
- A new sexual partner may have had a sexual pattern that included unsafe sex with high risk partners. They may not be honest if they desire sex with you or if they fear losing your interest in them.
- You and or your sex partner may have received a blood transfusion before the blood supply was tested and screened for contaminated blood.

As you can see, determining your level of risk may not be a simple matter. It is up to you to protect yourself. If you are in a committed relationship or married, the trust bond implies but does not guarantee full disclosure. Certainly we, as therapists, have helped many people struggle with this issue. Casual sex, adolescent/young adult sexual activity and new sexual partners do not lend themselves to full disclosure. Few people actually know if they have been exposed to AIDS. Those who know they have been exposed are aware that if they share this information with someone they want to have sex with, they may be turned down.

Although this guide may tell you more than you ever wanted to know about sex and AIDS, we believe that accurate information will help you determine your level of risk and better decide what course of action you need to take to feel safe and enjoy sex.

The Guide Is For Everyone

The Complete Guide to Safer Sex is both a general reference book on the sexual aspects of AIDS prevention and a "how to" book for people who want to create a safer and healthier sexual lifestyle. The book is written with the realization that people concerned about sex, health and AIDS come from a wide variety of backgrounds. Some of those are:

- People with varying degrees of sexual health knowledge to whom others turn for advice such as parents, teachers, health professionals or community leaders.
- People who enjoy rich sexual lives and want to know how to continue enjoying sexual pleasure without risking their health or the health of others.
- Individuals who are just beginning to explore sexuality at a time when safe sex techniques should be learned and practiced.
- People with AIDS, ARC, positive antibody test results, or who are at risk of HIV infection.
- People needing information for peace of mind or better communication and negotiation skills in order to create or maintain a safe sexual lifestyle.
- People who are not in danger in terms of sexual activity themselves, but who want to be well informed about AIDS and sexual risk reduction.

The Guide's Basic Premises

As sexologists, our special professional and ethical perspective has guided us in creating this book. Basically, *The Complete Guide to Safer Sex* rests upon the following premises:

1. **Sex can, and should, be the subject of serious, open and nonjudgemental discussion.** To facilitate healthy sexual choices, people need sexual knowledge, scientific facts and the ability to discuss sexual issues.
2. **Each individual is responsible for determining her or his own level of risk.**
3. **Each individual has the ability to create a satisfying safe sex lifestyle.** When people are provided with rich alternatives to unsafe sexual practices, they can create an effective risk reduction lifestyle which best suits their individual sexual, affectional and erotic needs.
4. **Everyone has a right to a good sex life.** Despite AIDS, everyone can enjoy a good sex life with safe sex techniques.
5. **AIDS prevention should not be dictated by law or government.** Sexuality is the most individualistic part of a person's life and has never been successfully legislated or controlled by force.

Taking A Nonjudgemental Approach

No matter what our background, we have all received conflicting messages about sexuality throughout our lives. Some messages are positive and supportive of sexuality, while many others are negative.

Undoubtedly, some who read this book will be in agreement with the common negative views; others will have no strong opinions or be confused; while still others will take the perspective that sex is a positive, spiritual, life-affirming expression which can be experienced without shame, guilt or intervention by others. It is not the intention of this book to sustain beliefs, challenge or persuade people regarding their attitudes toward sex or to make judgments about what people do sexually.

Our objective is to approach safe sex with total candor within the context of what people actually do sexually. People can get over sexual embarrassment, prudery and objections to the sexual practices of those different from themselves, but AIDS can not be prevented unless we improve our understanding of all sexual behavior and develop adequate sexual risk reduction strategies.

Sexual Enrichment— Reframing How We View Sex

Rather than rely on sexual denial to help people reduce the risk of AIDS, sexologists stress sexual enrichment as the best approach. Simply put, people are most able to change their sexual behavior when they increase their options for sexual fulfillment.

Finding ways to make high risk activities less risky without sacrificing enjoyment, we work toward helping people eroticize forms of protection such as the use of condoms, spermicides, latex gloves and other barriers to disease transmission.

In psychological terms, we stress **reframing sexuality**—letting go of our usual notions of what activities must or should take place for sex to be most satisfying. In the process of reframing sexuality, we open ourselves to exploring new sexual options including seldom used sexual activities or abstinence.

Dealing With AIDS And The Need For Safer Sex

When people first learn about the sexual ways AIDS can be transmitted, they often react in a variety of ways depending on the degree to which they personalize the risk. These include indifference, shock, fear, denial, anger, helplessness, numbness, depression, self-righteousness, indignation, hostility and/or vindictiveness. Some people experience a loss of sexual interest, others have increased sexual activity. Many people become despondent, feeling that sexual spontaneity has ended and mourn the loss of their sex life. As sexologists, we want to assure you that responsible sex can be erotic and satisfying. Despite the scaremongers, you do not have to give up sex.

How To Use This Book

Most people know very little about the range of common sexual behaviors. Even people who consider themselves very open and sexually sophisticated have strong reactions when they learn what others do sexually. Therefore, we urge the reader to remember certain points throughout reading the Guide in order to overcome any possible shock or discomfort:

- You do not have to like or dislike any part of the Guide nor do you have to follow any of the suggestions or exercises. YOU are in control and YOU have the personal right and obligation to create your own Safe Sex Lifestyle!
- If you find you are becoming uncomfortable, breathing deeply may help you relax.
- Feel free to skip around in the Guide to find the parts which most relate to your own life, sexual preferences, immediate needs and interests.
- If you are a parent or if you are reading the Guide to give advice to others, remember that you need to develop a relaxed, informed attitude in order to be most effective. Give yourself time to reflect on the information in the Guide with which you are unfamiliar.
- Finally, we invite you to explore and enjoy the Guide, and incorporate all the information and suggestions you want into your life.

Sex Is Fun!

Sex is fun is a concept that is threatened by the fear of AIDS and other STDs (sexually transmitted diseases). We have analyzed the scientific data concerning AIDS, with an agenda for preserving sexuality as a fun and healthy part of human contact and relationships.

The hysteria around AIDS has caused all of us to stop and wonder about our lifestyle and our motivation. Some individuals have used AIDS to promote their personal morality. "If you think and behave the way I tell you, you will be safe." We take a different stand, we think that you can be informed of the situation and make your own decisions. No person, government, religion, or other movement has been able to control people's sexuality. There is no reason to believe that AIDS will change that.

AIDS is not the first sexual plague that has befallen us. Syphilis and gonorrhea have also caused uncountable deaths and serious injuries to people. All the education and repression that was attempted did not stop the spread of these debilitating and sometimes deadly diseases. What controlled them eventually was medical science. The same will be true of AIDS. We can only slow the spread until medical science finds a cure or a vaccine or a treatment.

Our role then is not to stop people from being sexual. That is futile. We know that gratifying sexual expression is life enhancing. Our goal is to have people adopt risk reduction strategies (safe sex techniques) so that the

37

spread of human immunodeficiency virus (HIV) will be stemmed and give medical science a chance to figure out how to stop the transmission of the virus.

Not everyone who engages in sex with an infected person will contract the virus. Therefore, even if you have unsafe sex with an infected partner, you could but will not necessarily become infected yourself. Obviously, repeated unsafe contact with infected partners will raise your probability of contracting the virus considerably.

If everyone gave up all partnered sexual contacts, we believe that the quality of life would be decreased immensely. Also, people would tend to act out sexually in a compulsive manner, possibly in a violent manner, and the world would be a less happy place to live in. The treatment of depression would skyrocket and AIDS would still be spread by the desperate and guilt-laden acts of depressed individuals who just do not care anymore.

If we ask people who have chosen a lifestyle (or sexstyle) that is not monogamous to give it up and adopt a lifestyle that they have already rejected in some way, we should not be surprised by a high failure rate. Rather what we hope to do is show people how to reduce the risk of their chosen lifestyle, so that they can continue living their life as they wish.

CHAPTER 2
Thinking About AIDS

The History of AIDS

In 1978 a physician at NYU diagnosed a young gay man with Kaposi's sarcoma, a rare skin cancer usually seen only in older men of Mediterranean or African ancestry. He telephoned a colleague in Los Angeles, who also reported finding this rare cancer in young gay men. This was the initial awareness of existence of the disease that is now called AIDS. It was quickly noted that it affected the entire immune system and left the body vulnerable to "opportunistic infections" (OIs).

At the time, these OIs were primarily Kaposi's sarcoma (KS) and pneumocystis carinii pneumonia (PCP). By 1981, enough similar cases had developed for the Centers for Disease Control(CDC) to define a syndrome and establish a task force to study this new phenomenon.

Initially the disease appeared only to affect homosexual men. Thus, the syndrome was called "gay related immunodeficiency disease" or GRID. But doctors began reporting a similar condition among intravenous drug abusers in 1980, and by early 1982 it was apparent that the two groups were suffering from the same affliction. At the same time, other discernible groups manifested the condition—bisexual men, blood transfusion recipients, hemophiliacs, recent Haitian immigrants, sexual partners of people with AIDS and some of their newborn offspring. Accordingly, GRID was renamed the "acquired immunodeficiency syndrome" (AIDS).

As more cases developed scientists realized that there were many other opportunistic diseases associated with the syndrome. To differentiate between the official definition of AIDS, which included the almost always fatal OIs, from people with OIs that were thought to be less frequently fatal, the term "AIDS related condition" (ARC) was created. Though ARC is also know as "lesser AIDS," in reality ARC can be equally as serious as AIDS.

Competing theories about the etiology of AIDS (such as an overload of the immune system or rapid aging due to "living in the fast lane") gave way by 1983 to the idea that AIDS was caused by a specific transmissible agent, probably a virus. Early in 1984, a virus with several distinct forms was discovered which has been accepted by medical scientists as the cause or most significant factor in the development of AIDS.

It was evident early in the epidemic that AIDS was not spread through casual contact or even close association. Scientists found strong confirming evidence that AIDS was transmitted through blood or blood products and through intimate sexual contact. Sexual transmission was confirmed through tracing sexual partners. Thirteen of the first cases in southern California had engaged in sex with one another within 5 years of developing AIDS and one of those was eventually associated with 40 AIDS patients in 10 different parts of the country. Other clusters of homosexual partners who developed AIDS were also discovered.

During 1983–84, tracking of heterosexual contacts of AIDS patients established that AIDS can be sexually transmitted between men and women. By 1984, it seemed very clear that in Africa and Haiti AIDS was being transmitted through heterosexual sex. However, the exact mechanisms of how this occurred were not established. Indeed the presence of the virus in cervical/vaginal fluids was not confirmed until 1986.

Isolation of the AIDS virus in 1984 (now called HIV, human immunodeficiency virus) and the development of various tests that could identify both antibodies and the virus confirmed scientists' suspicion that there is a latency period during which most infected people are asymptomatic. That is, they look and feel healthy but are infected and may be infectious. Research also established that some people consistently test negative, never form antibodies to HIV, but have the virus and transmit it to others. They can also develop ARC and AIDS.

AIDS Antibody Testing

Testing for the AIDS virus has both scientific and political ramifications. Two separate tests, ELISA and

Western Blot, were developed to identify antibodies to HIV. The ELISA is a relatively inexpensive test, which has a higher incidence of false positives. The more accurate Western Blot is usually used to confirm a positive ELISA result. Even using both tests, a false positive or false negative result are still possible. It should be emphasized that all a positive antibody test result indicates is exposure to HIV and not that the person has or will develop AIDS.

Some governmental agencies have taken the position that it is every person's duty to be tested and inform others of their status. The CDC puts pressure on community health education programs to encourage voluntary testing and counseling. The armed forces and a few other agencies have mandatory testing.

Whether or not the test results provide an accurate assessment of a person's health status, there are personal, psychological and sociopolitical complications of a positive test result. In addition, positive or negative test results have not yet been shown to produce behavioral changes.

Rapid Transmission

One of the most distressing aspects of the history of AIDS is the rapidity with which the virus has been transmitted between people in the groups first hit—gay men, bisexual men, intravenous drug users, hemophiliacs, recipients of contaminated blood transfusions and their sex partners. In one study 24% were seropositive in 1978, but in 1984, 68% were seropositive.[1] It is common to see infection rates rise from 1% to 2% to 35% and more in just a few years. In the heterosexual population, while AIDS diagnosis has remained around 2%, this percentage is deceptive. The total number of heterosexual cases is increasing and the number of infected heterosexuals is unknown.

While scientists believe the virus is not particularly easily contracted we must ask how it has proliferated so rapidly. Major reasons given by researchers are:

1. Effective risk reduction programs are poorly funded, thus there are many infectious carriers who are not adequately aware of safe sex techniques.
2. The incubation period and healthy appearance of asymptomatic carriers create a false sense of security.
3. Many people do not believe they are at risk until they actually know people who are infected.
4. Over the years, people need constant support for safer sex practices or they fail to be safe every time.

The rate of infection for people outside of present highest risk groups and their sexual partners is estimated to be about 1/100,000. Accordingly, we all should be concerned and knowledgeable about AIDS and embark on a plan to ensure our personal safety.

Stages of Infection and Disease

The Centers For Disease Control proposed a classification some years ago which helps scientists categorize the whole range of phenomena which take place after a person is infected with HIV. Basically the stages are:

HIV I: Primary HIV Infection—Initial exposure and infection with the virus. This may or may not be accompanied by flu-like symptoms of fever, swollen lymph nodes, aching joints or muscles and diarrhea. Within the first six months, the body usually produces HIV antibodies.

HIV II: Asymptomatic seropositive—person feels healthy but is usually contagious and tests positive to the HIV antibody test.

HIV III: Persistent enlargement of the lymph nodes— (often in the armpits and back of neck) but otherwise remain relatively healthy.

HIV IV: Symptomatic HIV Infection—a general stage for all of the ARC and AIDS related opportunistic infections, tumors and neurological diseases. In the staging system, HIV IV can be subdivided into HIV IV: ARC autoimmune disease; HIV IV: ARC "minor" infections; HIV IV: Kaposi's sarcoma; HIV IV: lymphoma; and HIV IV: AIDS opportunistic infections.

The CDC continues to refine and reclassify stages of HIV disease and we can expect this process to continue for many years. The basic message is that HIV/AIDS is generally a slow, progressive process accompanied by a great variety of illnesses.

The Virus And How It Works

Several strains of the virus were discovered during 1984 and given different names: Human T-cell lymphotropic virus type III (HTLV—III), lymphadenopathy-associated virus (LAV), and AIDS-associated retrovirus (ARV). In 1986, after it became evident that HTLV-III, LAV and ARV were all isolates of the same virus group, the scientific community simplified the naming system by lumping all the strains under the term human immunodeficiency virus (HIV). In addition to the original three strains of HIV, two more have emerged. One which was discovered in West Africa is closely related to both a monkey AIDS virus (SRV-III) and to the LAV strain of HIV. It is called HIV II. The other has been isolated in South America and is called South American retrovirus (SARV). There are indications that other relatives of the HIV family also exist. (The general term for the AIDS virus is HIV.)

HIV belongs to a family of viruses, called retroviruses, which until now were only known in animals such as goats and horses. Among these animals, retroviruses cause brain or neurological deterioration and anemia. In 1985, it became evident that in addition to destroying the body's immune system and setting the stage for opportunistic infections, HIV also infects the nervous system of humans. Symptoms of advanced neurological damage from HIV are called "AIDS dementia."

The virus enters our body either as free virus present in body fluids or encapsulated in blood or other cells. Once inside a person's body, the virus attaches to cells and works its way inside. The virus may remain dormant for long periods of time and then, taking over the genetic material of the cell and making copies of itself, replicate in great numbers.

People may or may not catch more than one strain of HIV. However, the virus is constantly changing its structure within the body. This means that when infected people have sex or are exposed to the same strain of the virus at different times, they can contract or transmit variations of the same virus which may quickly attack new parts of their bodies. Thus even people who are infected must refrain from having unsafe sex with other people who are also infected.

Cofactors

HIV becomes much more deadly when certain other problems or "cofactors" are present. Some of these cofactors are the product of a lifestyle which weakens the immune system such as alcoholism, drug abuse, chronic stress and malnutrition. However, other cofactors are pathogens, particularly cytomegalovirus (CMV) and Epstein-Barr virus (EBV). Common sexually transmitted diseases—gonorrhea, syphilis, herpes, and candidiasis (yeast) create conditions which can greatly facilitate the transmission of the AIDS virus. The lesions which these pathogens create appear to be routes of transmission and in themselves can become so serious in advanced HIV disease that they can cause death.

Intestinal parasites such as amoebas are considered a possible cofactor of AIDS. These colonies of one-celled animals are transmitted most easily through contact with feces.

The Virus Is Very Fragile During Transmission

While presently there is no way to destroy HIV once it has successfully invaded a person's body, the virus is extremely easy to kill outside the body. For example, it can be killed instantly with nonoxynol-9 (a common ingredient of spermicides and some sexual lubricants), common soap and water, hydrogen peroxide, alcohol and bleach. All of these can be used in various ways to make sex safer. Some are for cleaning up and others are for preventing transmission during intercourse. In Chapter 4, we describe how to properly select, use and enjoy these helpers.

Developing An Attitude Toward AIDS You Can Live With

In Chapter 1, we mentioned the range of emotions which people experience when first learning the sexual risks of AIDS. Those who have been working in AIDS for a long time often see these emotions as aspects of a process—a process of loss with specific stages: a) indifference or denial, b) anger, c) bargaining, d) depression, and e) acceptance. In terms of the AIDS reality they might look something like this:

DENIAL: *"It's not my problem. I'm not in a high risk group—I'm more likely to get hit by lightning than get 'their' disease—all my partners are as healthy as I am."*

ANGER: *Is frequently characterized by trying to blame. "It's all 'their' fault—I'd like to round 'them' all up and maybe kill 'em!"*

BARGAINING: *"If I eat the right food, get enough sleep and go to the gym then I can do whatever I want sexually." "If I'm in love with my partner God won't punish us." "If I find a partner and we have a monogamous relationship I won't have to practice safe sex."*

DEPRESSION: *"I don't ever want to or can't have sex again." Frequently this stage is accompanied by a lower sexual drive or interest level.*

ACCEPTANCE: *"The crisis is not going to go away anytime soon. What are sex and risk reduction about in the Age of AIDS?"*

The reality of AIDS gives us all many reasons to grieve. These are very natural feelings and it is extremely important that we work through such emotional states rather than suppress or ignore them. If we deny the feelings which surround AIDS, they will surface in ways that are irrational and self-defeating. At best, some of the feelings help us to mobilize our personal resources to deal with the AIDS crisis and motivate us to change our personal risky activities. But more often, they are a hindrance to and a substitution for creating a healthy, happy, AIDS free lifestyle.

Shock, fear and denial will not prevent AIDS. Feelings of anger, helplessness, numbness and depression will not prevent AIDS. Only risk reduction can prevent AIDS. Let us honor and work through our emotions around AIDS. But even in the most difficult moments, let us also remember that risk reduction is our most effective defense against AIDS transmission. We should never use our feelings as an excuse to ignore or delay incorporating safe sex into our lives.

Indeed, as noted in the *acceptance* phase above, when the initial feelings pass and we begin to assess and explore the safer sexual options available in the Age of AIDS, we very often find that our lives return to normal and even improve. People who go on to construct a safe sex lifestyle often report an enhanced self concept, more respect for their partner or partners, loss of guilt feelings, and the enjoyment of sexual enrichment which comes from exploring new and safer sexual options.

Those who have gone through this process have much to offer people new to living in the Age of AIDS. These are a few of the successful strategies people take:

1. Approach AIDS prevention from a place of personal empowerment rather than from a place of fear and weakness. Make the AIDS challenge the chance you've always waited for to create the most rewarding lifestyle possible. Create a "new you." Consider

how you would like to be and then go about becoming that person.

2. Use the AIDS crisis as the impetus to create an overall health improvement plan—a holistic approach to health, life and happiness. Defeat the AIDS epidemic by becoming healthier than ever before. There are many ways to enhance our natural defenses against AIDS such as exercise, nutrition, stress reduction and adequate sleep.

3. Let go of fixed notions of how sex ought to be and approach it again with a willingness to learn totally new ways to experience and enjoy sexuality. As risk reduction becomes an adventure into new delights, feelings and ecstasy, unsafe sex becomes less important. Indeed, for many people risky sex becomes a bore.

4. Seek out the company of other people also into preventing AIDS and making themselves happier, fuller people in the process. It's tremendously helpful and great fun to compare strategies, ideas, success stories.

5. Avail yourself of community resources that can help you achieve your objectives. Working with groups dedicated to AIDS prevention through personal growth and change can speed up the process immensely.

6. Develop a support group to help you through the rough times. And remember that helping other members is a rewarding growth experience, too.

7. Be willing to learn from others whose lifestyle,

sexual orientation and other characteristics are different from your own. We all have a great deal to learn from one another. Be willing to share and learn from gays, bisexual men, women, heterosexuals, rubber fetishists, members of the S/M community, phone sex experts and others. We are all in this AIDS problem together and each of us have a contribution to make in stopping the spread of the virus.

8. We can have a happy, hot, wholesome, full life in the Age of AIDS. Indeed, a better, healthier life and a richer sex life are wonderful ways to get revenge on the evils of AIDS.

CHAPTER 3
Safe Sex Guidelines

Introduction

In this chapter we will:

- Examine the importance of creating layers of risk reduction in our sex lives.
- Look at basic safe sex guidelines.
- Learn why we must each take personal responsibility for creating our own personal guidelines.
- Review pertinent medical and epidemiological information to help us in this task.

The Most Basic Prevention Concepts

Safe sex guidelines change as more is known about AIDS transmission, but the most enduring advice is: **Do not exchange body fluids.** It's not sex that causes AIDS, but the migration of the virus from one person to another. As indicated, this is most easily accomplished when the infected blood, semen or cervical/vaginal secretions of one person enter the body of another. Other secretions which often contain HIV are saliva, tears, sweat and urine. However, under most conditions, transmission through contact with these substances is considered difficult or unlikely.

In 1991, a new route of HIV transmission was reported; from the skin of the penis to the vaginal, anal and oral mucosa and from the mucosa to the penis. This type of transmission is called "dendritic transmission." Basically, since 1987 there has been a growing body of evidence that Langerhan cells in the skin (particularly the genitals, rectum and mouth) are extremely vulnerable to HIV infection. These cells are part of the "dendritic system" which ordinarily helps the body fight off infections that come into contact with the skin or mucosal lining of the body cavities. However, in the case of AIDS, these cells become easily infected producing more AIDS virus than any other cells in the body.

Scientists feel that infection takes place during unprotected intercourse. During intercourse, aided by the body's moist internal environment, the abundant virus in the infected skin of the penis or the mucosal lining migrates from one person to another. At present, we do not know how often or easily this takes place, but the bottom line is to be safe use barrier protection for all penetration sex.

Creating Layers of Risk Reduction

What's safe, safer, safest?
What's risky, riskier, riskiest?
How does something safe become risky?
How does something risky become safe?

A sexual act includes many distinct activities (e.g. touching, kissing, genital contact). Each of these activities have different possible risks attached to them and call for different risk reduction strategies. Risk reduction strategies can be thought of as layers of protection against contact with HIV. It is important to have different strategies available for the same activity and it may be wise to use more than one layer of protection at the same time. The more types of risk reduction we incorporate into sex, the safer we will be.

If you do not come into contact with your partner's body fluids, you will not come in contact with HIV. For some people this prohibition is so great that they will not trust any safe sex precaution, and refrain from all sex. This is an overreaction and not necessary. Exactly where you drawn the line, what behaviors you think are too dangerous, and what precautions or lack of precautions too risky is an individual decision for each of us to make with the aid of the latest scientific research. We call this process "developing levels of risk reduction."

Before we explore what this really means, we need to put our reactions to AIDS into perspective. Most of us endanger our lives everyday by getting into a car and driving somewhere. The chances of being killed in a car accident are much greater than dying from AIDS. Yet, few of us are so terrified of driving that we refuse to leave the relative safety of our homes. Instead we go through a variety of risk reduction strategies to reduce the chance of being involved in an accident. These include wearing seat belts, appropriately servicing the car, not speeding, not driving under the influence of alcohol or drugs, becoming a vigilant driver looking out for the other guy, etc. This brand of defensive driving is analogous to safe sex.

Taking the analogy further, not everyone does everything. Some people speed, some people don't wear seat belts all the time, some people do some things to decrease their chances of getting into an accident, but not everything. The same is true of safe sex. Not everyone is willing to take the same risks or change the same behaviors, because of the differences in their priority system.

For example, anal intercourse has been shown to be a behavior that has particularly high correlation with contracting the virus. If you do not particularly like anal intercourse, it may be easiest for you to give up the behavior completely. If you have found that anal intercourse is a particularly fun and pleasurable behavior, you may want to search for ways to make it safer. You may be willing to tolerate a higher risk by doing the behavior in a safer way than just giving up and doing it unsafely.

For example, you can engage in anal intercourse with the inserter wearing a condom. It might be even safer if the inserter wears two condoms. You might use extra nonoxynol-9 lubricant. You might find a partner that you can be monogamous with, and after appropriate screening tests live a monogamous lifestyle. It is important to note that none of these suggestions is foolproof, and all carry somewhat more risk than eliminating the behavior from your sex life altogether.

Therefore, the level of risk reduction that you use is an individual decision based on your lifestyle and desires. Each of us will make an individual decision about what amount of risk we are willing or unwilling to take. To the extent that we make an adequate decision, the transmission of this disease will decrease.

The risk inherent in every situation can be reduced in some way. It is probably foolish for anyone to say that they will be perfect. Most of us have problems staying on diets or keeping to anything perfectly. Situations present themselves in a way that is unexpected. The result is lapses and slips.

If you are going to take part in an unsafe behavior, then it is to your advantage to expose yourself to as little risk as possible. For example, if you run out of condoms then you could withdraw prior to orgasm. You could use the plastic wrap used to wrap leftovers. Neither of these is recommended nor considered a safe sex technique, but it is clearly better than doing nothing.

Therefore, you always have some control over how safe a situation is. That is what is meant by risk reduction behavior. You may have decided that you would not take the risk of sharing saliva, but if you slip then gargling afterwards with a mouthwash may be better than nothing at all. If mouthwash was not available, then just gargling with salt water or even plain water is better than nothing. The idea is to reduce the chance that the virus will get into your system.

Some Poor Strategies

Let's talk for a minute about what has been suggested as risk reduction strategies, but are **not recommended** (at least by the authors of this book) anymore:

Know your sex partners: While a good idea, it really only asks that your partner lie to you. If someone who has been involved in high risk behavior knows what your criteria are, then lying is the only way s/he will have a sexual experience with you. You are asking to be lied to, which does not help the communication process that you hope will exist with your new partner.

Be monogamous: Again this is a set up for someone to lie to you. If you believe that your partner is monogamous and s/he is not, then you are being un-knowingly exposed. Obviously, there are monogamous couples out there, but you need to be careful about just assuming that your partner is monogamous. It is also important to recognize that if your partner commits an indiscretion, s/he may be afraid to tell you because of the ramifications (splitting up, divorce, lack of trust in the future, etc.). While negative reaction to a partner's nonmonogamy is understandable, that reaction might have just the effect you are hoping to avoid—further lies and continuation of unsafe sexual practices.

This especially applies to those people who have attempted to deal with AIDS by only having sex within a group of friends, after everyone has been screened for the virus. If someone in that group has an outside sexual contact, then s/he is under considerable pressure not to reveal it, because doing so would alienate him/her from his/her support group and sexual partners.

A negative antibody test means it is safe: First, there are still both false negatives (test says you are not infected, but you are) and false positives (test says you are infected, but you are not). Additionally, an HIV infection can take several months to produce the antibodies which make test results turn positive, and you may still be infectious during that time. Further, you may have contracted the virus since you took the test.

Reduce your number of sex partners: While this is not bad advice, one infected partner is all you need. You can do any sexual act with any number of partners and not contract the virus, as long as all those partners are virus free. Reducing the number of partners does reduce your risk of coming into contact with an infected partner, but it really depends on your choice of sex partners.

Be abstinent: While the strategy of refraining from sex with others is one way to stop the transmission of AIDS, it does not work for everyone. It is an often simplistic reaction and a way of not thinking or talking about sex. However, suppressing sexuality is a virtual impossibility for most people and it *does not* make sex go away!

We encounter people who abstain from sex for a period of time and then go on sexual binges—binges in which they are totally unprepared to practice safe sex and wind up engaging in extremely risky activities. This then gives way to feelings of extreme fear and guilt followed by the cycle of abstinence and bingeing again.

How Safe Sex Guidelines Are Structured

It is common to divide risk reduction guidelines into three categories:

- **Safe or very low risk** activities which present the least likelihood of HIV transmission;
- **Probably safe or possibly risky** activities which contain elements of possible risk or about which there is insufficient knowledge and information; and
- **Unsafe** activities which have been clearly linked to HIV transmission.

Unfortunately, no one, including us, can state definitely what to do and not to do to prevent HIV transmission. The safe sex guidelines of different agencies vary and agencies change guidelines as new information becomes available. But while there is a legitimate disagreement between professionals and groups on what is safe and what is not, the following list is accepted by most authorities and the authors of the Guide.

Our Brand of Safe Sex Guidelines

Safe or Very Low Risk

- **Sexual fantasies** of any kind
- **Sex talk** (romantic, simply informational or "talking dirty")
- **Flirting**

- **Hugging**
- **Social (dry) kissing**
- **Phone sex**
- **Bathing together** (including erotic bathing)
- **Body massage** (including erotic and nongenital oral massage)
- **Smelling bodies and body fluids**
- **Tasting our own body fluids**
- **Body licking** (on healthy, clean skin)
- **Consensual exhibitionism and Voyeurism** (showing off and watching)
- **Masturbation** (mutual or solitary—penile, vaginal, clitoral)—Do not use a partner's body fluids as a lubricant.
- **Using personal sex toys**
- **S&M games** (without bruising or bleeding)
- **Sensuous feeding**
- **Sex movies, videos and tapes**
- **Erotic books and magazines**
- **Live sexual entertainment**

Probably Safe, Possibly Risky

- **French kissing**
- **Fellatio without ejaculation** (safer with a condom)
- **Fellatio with ejaculation wearing a condom**
- **Cunnilingus** (oral-vaginal sex, safer with a latex barrier and/or spermicide)
- **Peno-vaginal intercourse with condom** (safer with spermicide, safer yet when combined with a cervical barrier—diaphragm, cap or sponge)

- **Digital-anal sex with glove** (assplay with latex or plastic glove)
- **Anal intercourse with condom** (safer to withdraw before ejaculation)
- **Anilingus with latex** (anal-oral sex, rimming through a rubber dam or condom)
- **Contact with urine** (golden showers or water sports on unbroken skin)

Unsafe

- **Vaginal intercourse without a condom**
- **Anal intercourse without a condom**
- **Swallowing semen**
- **Receiving semen vaginally**
- **Unprotected oral-anal contact**
- **Unprotected manual-anal intercourse** (fist fucking without a latex glove)
- **Unprotected manual-vaginal intercourse** (fisting the vagina without a latex glove.
- **Sharing menstrual blood**
- **Sharing needles or blood while piercing or shooting drugs**

  Risk increases with the number of partners in unprotected activities! Risk increases when people are drunk or high on drugs!

Risk Factors Change Situationally

Safe sex guidelines are a *general guide* but the *risk factors change situationally*. You must consider the particulars of every sexual encounter in order to use the guidelines correctly. For example, if you or your partner have cuts or broken skin, then even low risk activities become riskier and more precaution is wise. If you or your partner have a raw throat, sore in your mouths or bleeding gums, then oral activities are probably more risky.

Oral lesions, which are often sexually transmitted AIDS cofactors (i.e. herpes I & II and CMV ulcers) are extremely common among people who are HIV positive and symptomatic.

Genitals which are dry or irritated can present increased risk. Other factors include how you actually do the sexual act! For example, untrimmed fingernails can make any digital intercourse somewhat riskier. Unplanned opportunistic sex may increase your level of risk as it prompts you to throw caution to the wind. Your general health is a factor in your ability to resist and fight any infection including HIV.

Remember, your sexual pattern is unique and personal. Only you can determine the level of risk in your overall sexual pattern or any specific sexual situation.

Personal Responsibility

Being actively involved in creating personal guidelines is exhilarating to some people, but others would be much happier if the guidelines were just handed to them. However, because we are only beginning to understand HIV transmission and because each sexual encounter requires unique judgements, taking personal responsibility is absolutely necessary.

It is obviously up to you to be as informed as possible and *make your own decisions based on the known facts*. This process is continuous because scientific understanding about HIV transmission is constantly being updated. The following review of pertinent scientific research will provide a range of opinions which will enable you to make informed decisions. It is a foundation from which to evaluate new findings.

Scientific Basis of the Guidelines

Scientists have been studying how AIDS is transmitted since 1981. Their research has focused upon the possibility of:

a) Transmission in ordinary social situations
b) Transmission within households where a person is infected with HIV, has ARC or has AIDS
c) Transmission in a hospital setting
d) Transmission by insects or parasites
e) Sexual transmission
f) Transmission in utero or through lactation
g) Transmission through blood transfusions

Lack of Casual Transmission

Again, AIDS is not transmitted through casual contact such as shaking hands, hugging, social kissing, sneezing, coughing, face-to-face conversation, touching or sitting close to an infected person. Researchers point out that if this were the case, the epidemic would be much larger and wider spread in the general population.[1]

Lack of Household Transmission

There is strong evidence that even in close living arrangements, HIV is not spread. A study of 101 people in AIDS households found that the virus was not transmitted to other household members despite sharing the toilet, bath, shower, towels, nail clippers, combs, clothes, eating utensils, eating plates, drinking glasses, beds, toothbrushes, or even razors. The same study showed no transmission from hugging, kissing on the cheek or kissing on the lips.[2] These findings have been corroborated by continuing research in the United States, Europe and Africa.

Lack of Transmission Via Insects

The possibility of HIV transmission by insects and parasites has not been entirely ruled out, though there are studies which strongly indicate that insects are not transmitting the infection.

Inferential evidence from African research indicates that body lice and head lice do not transmit HIV. Close living quarters and sleeping habits frequently result in the same colony of lice infecting all members of a household, yet HIV transmission remains limited to sexual partners within households and children newly born to infected parents.

One of the most rigorous studies of mosquitoes and AIDS was conducted in Belle Glade, Florida. This area has been a focus of national attention because it has an extremely high number of AIDS cases and because these cases are primarily heterosexual.

The research team looked at patterns of AIDS distribution in neighborhoods of Belle Glade and nearby towns. They interviewed and tested people living in neighborhoods with high numbers of AIDS cases for the presence of HIV antibodies AND the presence of other viruses commonly transmitted by mosquitoes. The team found no evidence of transmission of HIV by mosquitoes. The study did show that HIV in Belle Glade is primarily transmitted through contaminated needles and sexual contact with infected intravenous drug users.[3] Indeed, a follow-up study found more seronegative people had been infected with common mosquito viruses than seropositives.[4]

Safety in Hospital Settings

HIV-infected patients are handled without extra measures under most circumstances in hospitals (feeding, bathing, massaging). However, medical personnel are advised to wear latex gloves, goggles and masks when handling body fluids. They are also advised to wash and change clothes immediately when there are spills and splashes of infected materials and to clean all surfaces with disinfectant. Soiled bedding and clothing of AIDS patients are to be doubled bagged and labeled. These procedures and more are regularly published by Centers for Disease Control (CDC) and various medical journals, but essentially have remained unchanged since early in the epidemic.[5]

However, even with these precautions, accidents do happen and some healthcare workers have been exposed numerous times during their work. In February 1985, CDC reported on 361 health care workers who had been exposed. The types of exposure were: needlestick injuries (68%); mucosal exposures (13%), cuts with sharp instruments (10%), and contamination of open skin lesions with potentially infected body fluids (9%). Eighty-eight percent of the exposures were to blood or serum; 6% to saliva; 2% to urine; and the remaining 4% to other body fluids of unknown sources. Postexposure care varied considerably. Forty-eight percent of exposed healthcare workers received either no specific treatment or local wound care only, while 35% received immunoglobulin either alone or in combination with other treatment. Of these injured medical personnel, only two became infected with AIDS.[6] As of May 1986, only four healthcare workers out of over 1,000 who reported accidental exposure to HIV has become infected from their work place. In 1987 a major review of hospital transmission concluded that occupational transmission of HIV will remain uncommon. This conclusion has been upheld by continued monitoring.

Sexual Transmission

To understand sexual transmission, scientists:

1. Take retrospective sex histories, asking people what they did before becoming infected with HIV.
2. Conduct prospective studies following the sexual activities and health status of large groups of people at risk for HIV infection to see what statistically significant factors can be discovered.
3. Compare risk groups and routes of transmission in different parts of the world in order to understand the various ways the virus might be transmitted.
4. Conduct laboratory studies on infected body fluids and tissue to ascertain how the virus is sexually transmitted.
5. Study transmission using animal models, usually monkeys or chimpanzees.

In reviewing their findings, we will concentrate on HIV transmission through contact with the penis, mouth, vagina and anus.

Penile Transmission

The role of transmission through infected semen is well known, but few researchers have studied the factors which increase the risk of HIV being transmitted to the penis. One study suggests, however, that a dry, raw, inflamed or diseased urethra or penis puts men at considerable added risk.[7]

With the growing knowledge about dendritic transmission, it appears that when the penis is in contact with the mucosa of infected body cavities, transmissions can occur. Animal studies indicate that this can take place through the skin of the shaft of the penis, but particularly through the urethra, the head of the penis and the foreskin.[8]

Oral Transmission

Early in the AIDS epidemic, medical researchers theorized that the agent which caused AIDS was not easily transmitted by oral contact. They reached this conclusion stating that if the agent were easily transmitted orally, the entire population would be randomly coming down with AIDS instead of clearly defined risk groups. Accordingly, many early AIDS prevention guidelines placed French kissing in the SAFE category and unprotected oral sex in the POSSIBLY SAFE category.

However, in February 1984 scientists reported a case of AIDS which seems to have been transmitted through kissing.[9] Shortly afterwards, the same researchers found HIV in the saliva of infected people. They noted that retroviruses are sometimes transmitted in other animals through saliva and cautioned people at risk to avoid direct contact with saliva.[10]

This led most agencies to move French kissing from SAFE to the POSSIBLY SAFE category. Some advised people to avoid French kissing all together or any other activity involving saliva. All agencies advised people to take overall oral health into consideration before French kissing. Oral sex without swallowing ejaculate was thought to be POSSIBLY SAFE and oral sex WITH swallowing ejaculate was moved to the UNSAFE category. Most AIDS educators began to advise the use of condoms during oral sex.

In June of 1985, Canadian researchers published results of the Vancouver Lymphadenopathy-AIDS Study, an ongoing epidemiological study of over 700 homosexual men, which indicated that oral sex did not transmit HIV. They stated, "Even swallowing semen did not appear to confer any increased risk."[11]

A clinical report from the U.S. bolstered the initial results of the Vancouver epidemiological study. Researchers found that of 73 patients infected with HIV, the virus was detected only in the saliva of one man, a patient who had a serious opportunistic infection in his throat. These investigators concluded that oral transmission was difficult and probably unlikely.[12]

In February 1986, the Vancouver researchers stated their findings more strongly in a letter to The Lancet, the highly respected British medical journal. They found that of 99 seronegative men who continued to engage in receptive anal intercourse, 36 (35%) became seropositive in less than two years. However, of 21 seronegative men whose main outlet was oral sex, only 1 became seropositive. They concluded:

> The sexual practices of the 21 men we studied, the number of their partners, and the prevalence of HTLV-III seropositivity in homosexual men in Van-

couver (at least 35%) combine to suggest that during the observation period these men received frequent oral exposure to HTLV-III. Yet only 1 man seroconverted and this probably happened through insertive anal intercourse, a known mode of transmission. Our findings corroborate the lack of oral transmission of HTLV-III.[13]

In March of 1986, laboratory research conducted by Harvard University strengthened the position that HIV is hard to transmit orally. Importantly, their findings contradicted the earlier clinical report that HIV is rare in the saliva of infected people. In fact, the Harvard researchers found that 70% of their AIDS patients and 93% of the ARC patients had AIDS antibodies in their saliva. **However, their conclusion was the same.** The difference in finding the virus was due to methods of testing. When the Harvard researchers used immunoglobulin (Ig) tests instead of blood antibody tests, they found abundant HIV in their patients' saliva, but the virus had been neutralized by immunoglobulin A (IgA). They concluded that the immunoglobulin in saliva might protect the body from oral transmission of HIV.[14]

At the 1986 International Conference on AIDS in Paris, several papers were presented which supported the position that HIV is not easily transmitted orally. One of the most important, **The Multi-Center AIDS Collaborative Study** (MACS) looked at over 2000 men during a six month period. Not one of the 213 men who refrained from anal sex but continued to have oral sex became seropositive. However, 3.5% of 1,637 males who had anal sex with some partners and 12.2% of 246 men who had anal sex with most or all of their partners became seropositive. The researchers concluded that refraining from anal sex even while continuing oral intercourse can significantly reduce the risk of infection with HIV and that transmission of HIV through other than anal practices may be rare.[15]

Also presented was an extremely important case study of bites and scratches in which 188 health care workers in contact with an ARC patient hemophiliac were studied. The man had been brain damaged due to an automobile accident. In a two-year period while he had typical manifestations of ARC, he inflicted bites and scratches on 30 health care workers causing skin puncture wounds and residual scars. His mouth was frequently full of saliva and blood, his fingernails soiled with semen, feces and urine. Extensive immune evaluation was carried out on all personnel six months after skin trauma. All 188 were normal and there were no significant differences between the bite and casual contact groups. All persons bitten or scratched were HIV antibody negative. Thus, the researchers concluded, the risk of transmission of HIV from bites and scratches under similar conditions should be very low.[16]

Just as many people were becoming convinced that French kissing and oral sex were safe or very low risk and when some AIDS educators were lowering the barriers, the Harvard scientists repeated their good news about IgA possibly preventing oral transmission but also issued a warning:

The frequency of IgA deficiency in the general population is 1 in 450. Several cases of IgA deficiency have been described in patients with AIDS. . . . If IgA antibodies to HIV prove to be neutralizing, HIV may be transmissible by saliva that lacks IgA. Further research will help clarify this.[17]

Another researcher cautioned researchers about the hastiness of reaching conclusions with existing data:

Recent contributors to The Lancet have incautiously reached the conclusion that HTLV-III/LAV is not transmitted orally or via saliva, and this conclusion has been incorporated into guidelines for safe sex aimed at reducing the risk of AIDS. Most people identified as having been infected sexually by HTLV-III are presumed to have contracted the virus through a genitally linked route, a presumption that is probably correct most of the time. However, genital contact is often preceded by erotic kissing, and it is a mistake to assume that infection always results from the genital contact rather than the oral, unless these two routes have been convincingly teased apart.[18]

Research about the role of kissing in HIV transmission continues to generate controversy. The general rule remains that when the mouths of the individuals kissing are healthy, kissing is safe. However, an often overlooked problem is that people who are in advanced stages of HIV disease (ARC or AIDS) overwhelmingly have chronic bleeding conditions in their mouths. Many of these conditions are viral STD infections associated with

HIV transmission or progression to AIDS: for example, herpes I and II, CMV and EBV. This is why oral contact is in the **Probably Safe—Possibly Risky** category.

Peno-Vaginal Transmission

In the United States, the number of people infected by HIV transmission between men and women is low compared to HIV transmitted between men. It is important to remember, however, that while the percentage has stayed the same (about 3%), as the total number of cases increases the number of heterosexual cases also increases.

We will provide information on many forms of vaginal sex at the end of this section. However, we will limit our exploration of vaginal transmission primarily to peno-vaginal intercourse, the activity about which most is known. The most recent summary overview is an excellent article by Nancy J. Alexander, "Sexual Transmission and Human Immunodeficiency Virus: Virus Entry into the Male and Female Genital Tract." Published in the journal of Fertility and Sterility 1990 (54) 1:1–18.

HIV has been repeatedly cultured from cervical/vaginal tissues and fluids.[20] The amount of virus increases when women become sexually stimulated.[21] Although the amount of HIV is much lower than in sperm, vaginal transmission has been documented by research. HIV transmission between men and women was first recognized in the United States in 1983[22] and peno-vaginal intercourse is a known route of AIDS transmission in Haiti and Africa.[23]

In most U.S. cases resulting from sex between men

and women, one of the partners was a member of an already existing high risk group. African research also indicates that vaginal transmission of HIV is probably slower and less efficient than other forms of transmission. However, studies in Africa and Haiti consistently report that while contaminated needles and blood transfusions are important factors, vaginal intercourse is considered the main route of heterosexual transmission.[24] [25]

Some people think culture and genetics make the experience of heterosexual Africans so unique that it has no relevance to HIV transmission between men and women elsewhere. This is not true. But how common is bi-directional heterosexual HIV infection and how certain are we that vaginal intercourse is the route of transmission? The routes are not entirely clear or uncontradictory, but unprotected coitus with an infected partner is definitely high risk. Our best guess approximates the risk of pregnancy or gonorrhea, which is one in three. [See APPENDIX]

Instead of asking whether AIDS virus is transmitted vaginally, scientists are now focusing intently upon the question "What factors enhance the possibility that HIV will be transmitted." A leading hypothesis is that active sexually transmitted diseases and other genital infections play a major role by breaking down the protective walls of the vagina and allowing HIV to enter the blood. It is felt that such infections also facilitate transmission of HIV from women to men by creating lesions of the penis and destroying the mucosal lining of the urethra.[26]

Other Forms of Vaginal Sex

Oral-vaginal sex has not been proven as a route of AIDS transmission but the risk is thought to fall somewhere in the same range as other oral sexual activities.

Masturbation of the clitoris and vagina by a partner as a route of transmission has not been studied though there is speculation that if the female genitals are irritated and/or the partner has cuts, sores or abrasions on the hands, or if semen and vaginal fluids are mixed, HIV transmission is possible.

Most researchers have not generally acknowledged that vaginal fisting, inserting a hand in the vagina, exists. Accordingly, neither women with AIDS nor their partners have been asked regularly about this activity. It is assumed unsafe, but much less risky if an examination glove is worn.

Since anal douching before or after sex is linked to higher risk of AIDS because it creates small tears, it is possible that vaginal douching is also unsafe. However, vaginal douching and HIV transmission has not been studied.

Because sharing toys anally has been shown to place partners at higher risk, sharing toys vaginally is also considered risky but has not been studied.

Anal Transmission

From very early in the AIDS crisis, there has been strong evidence that unprotected anal intercourse, especially receptive anal sex, is a major way that HIV is transmitted. Inserting the hand in the rectum (fisting) has also been associated with HIV transmission in some studies, and to some extent, oral-anal contact (rimming) has also been implicated.[27]

While anal transmission of HIV is a well known fact, there is a great deal of misinformation on the topic. Remember these truths about anal sex and AIDS:

- The virus also is transmitted in many ways—not just receptive anal intercourse.
- In anal intercourse, both the inserter and his partner are at risk.
- Fisting is risky for both partners.
- Many anal activities are safe. Anal self-pleasuring, assplay with a latex or plastic glove, using clean personal toys and rimming through a latex barrier are all ways to play safely.

Conclusion

While safe sex is the most important deterrent we have against HIV transmission, it is not known if these guidelines are completely adequate or if they are overly cautious. The most important guideline remains ***don't share body fluids, and use barrier protection every time there is anal, vaginal or oral penetration sex.*** Sometimes determining what activities prevent such exchange is easy, but sometimes it is difficult. We have not covered all sexual activities in this chapter but we have discussed the most researched behaviors to date and hope we have provided you with enough information to assess your own personal level of risk. In the following chapters, we will provide many techniques designed to minimize your risk and enhance your sex life.

CHAPTER 4
All About Condoms, Lubricants, Spermicides and Other Helpers

In this chapter we will:

- Look at condoms and other latex products in greater depth.
- Share basic information about lubricants and spermicides.
- List common products which can help stop the virus.

The chapter is intended, of course, as sex education—not medical advice.

Condoms

Condoms are an extremely important weapon in the war against AIDS and other sexually transmitted diseases. To make best use of these "little soldiers of love" we must choose the right kind, use them properly, and learn how to enjoy them.

The instructions for proper condom use provided here are synthesized from a number of scientific articles while the section on condom enjoyment comes from discussions with thousands of condom users, hints from the scientific journals and personal exploration.

Before proceeding, let us stress the point once more that while condoms are extremely important for safeguarding our sexual health, they are not a total solution to AIDS prevention. Obviously the more layers of risk reduction we use and the healthier lives we lead, the greater chances are that we will survive the AIDS epidemic.

Are Condoms Effective Against AIDS?

When properly used, condoms create a strong protective barrier to the spread of many sexually transmitted diseases (STDs). Early in the AIDS epidemic, scientists theorized that condoms would help prevent AIDS because the virus that causes the disease is roughly the size of herpes and other viruses which are unable to penetrate latex; further, neither air nor water can pass through condoms even though their molecules are a 1,000 times smaller than such viruses. In 1985, a rigorous laboratory study demonstrated that AIDS virus could not get through condoms. Although there are important differences between laboratory studies and clinical tests, sexologists and others in the AIDS prevention field are more convinced than ever that condoms play an extremely important role in preventing the spread of AIDS. Continuing studies of people at high risk for HIV infection who use condoms regularly are confirming this conviction.

Condoms also help prevent several of the opportunistic infections and cofactors associated with AIDS. For example, they help stop genital transmission of candidasis (yeast infections), cytomegalovirus (CMV), Epstein-Barr virus (EBV), herpes, chancroid, gonorrhea, and syphilis.

How To Use Condoms Correctly

Practice Makes Perfect!

Instructions for condom use are simple but must be followed carefully. The main reason condoms fail is incorrect use. They seldom leak or break due to faulty manufacture.

1. Keep a convenient supply of condoms in a cool, dry place for "every time" use.
2. Do not test condoms by inflating or stretching them.
3. Use condoms *EVERY* time you have intercourse, even for oral sex.
4. Open the package carefully. Rough handling can damage condoms, especially if nails are long or jagged.
5. With your thumb and forefinger, gently press any air out of the receptacle tip at the closed end before putting on the condom—air bubbles can cause condoms to break. Plain-ended condoms require about a half inch free at the tip to catch the ejaculation. A dab of lubricant in the tip will solve the air problem and greatly increase sensation.

6. Unroll the condom so that it covers the entire penis. If a man is uncircumcised, the foreskin should be pulled back before covering the head with the condom. Fitting an erect penis with a condom insures the best fit, but if the penis is soft, be sure to unroll the entire condom down to the base as the organ hardens. If the condom does not fit completely to the bottom of a man's penis, he should be careful not to insert beyond the condom base as this can cause the condom to come off.

7. Use plenty of water-soluble lubricant on the outside of the condom and on the vagina or anus before entry. Areas that are too dry can pull condoms off and tear them as well. Oil-based lubricants like baby oil, cold cream, Crisco and Vaseline cause condoms to quickly break.

8. Hold onto the base of the condom when necessary so the condom won't slip off. If the penis is getting soft, or if a partner is very tight, the condom may tend to slip. Certain sexual positions also tend to cause slipping. For example when a woman is sitting on top of a man, the lips of her vagina can lift off the condom. Holding the base of the condom will solve the problem.

9. After ejaculation, hold onto the condom around the base to avoid spilling the contents or losing the condom inside a partner. Withdraw gently.

10. Throw used condoms away! They should not be used more than once. NEVER go from one person to another without changing condoms.

Picking The Condom That's Right For You

When looking for the "right" condom the main thing to do is **experiment!!!** Try out lots of different kinds using low risk activities such as masturbation, and rubbing between the thighs or breasts. Be sure to **break some** so you know how much stress they can take and what it feels like when one is torn.

Latex or Natural Condoms?

Although some users prefer condoms made from the appendix of sheep, latex provides much better protection. The animal fiber condoms have walls of unequal thickness and sometimes leak. **ALWAYS** use good latex condoms!

Wet or Dry?

Lubricated condoms do not break as easily as unlubricated ones. They also give a moist natural sexual feeling to the skin that the dry powdered ones do not. This creates greater sensation for the wearer.

Condoms are lubricated with gels or silicone-based products. Gels coat prophylactics unevenly inside the package, while silicone products lubricate all parts of the condom equally. The silicone coating is less gooey when the package is opened and the thorough wetness means they are less likely to break from grabbing on dry spots during use.

Some condoms are lubricated with nonoxynol-9, a

substance which kills AIDS virus in test tube studies. These are advertised as having a spermicidal lubricant. Important considerations in choosing to use such condoms are:

- They may provide local protection against AIDS in case the condom breaks, leaks or spills; however,
- Nonoxynol-9 lubricated condoms have only been tested for vaginal intercourse. Accordingly, some using them for anal intercourse may wish to put the condom on and then wipe off the outside so as to have added protection on the inside of the condom without using it on anal tissue; and
- Some people find nonoxynol-9 mildly irritating. Nonoxynol-9 products should be tried out first, using low risk activities before taking a chance on becoming chapped and creating a possible route for infection. Problems with irritation can usually be solved by simply changing spermicidal brands.

Should They Fit Like a Glove?

With condoms, *exact size isn't everything!* Latex hugs and stretches to fit many sizes. Condoms which fit snugly slightly constrict the superficial veins of the penis making erections harder and orgasms more intense. Sex therapists often suggest this approach to men who are having trouble maintaining an erection during sex. Condoms with more room at the top allow the end of the condom to move and thus create more sensation. Length is not critical so long as the condom goes all the way to the base of the penis and people are careful during intercourse not to penetrate beyond where the condom ends. Shop around with fun as well as safety in mind.

Some people have tremendous fear that condoms will come off during sex. Further, because of the variety in penis shapes and sizes a few men do have a serious problem finding a condom brand which will stay on. There is an excellent brand of condoms on the market, *Mentor Contraceptives*, which has an adhesive on the inside that seals to the skin. Sometimes referred to as "synthetic skin" this particular condom has the ability to shrink or stretch if a man's penis becomes softer or harder during sex while staying firmly in place.

Is Thicker Stronger?

Some condoms are thicker than others but modern production techniques have led to condoms of reduced thickness without sacrificing essential strength required by federal standards.

More important than thickness for strength is the *age* of the condom and the way it is treated before and during use. Condoms have a shelf life of 5 years under optimal conditions but begin to deteriorate slowly after 2½ years. Buy from a distributor who has a good turnover. Condoms also age quickly from heat, strong light and rough treatment. Don't leave them in the sun or keep them in car glove compartments. And don't keep them in billfolds for long periods.

What About Different Shapes?

Condoms with receptacle tips to catch the ejaculate are recommended over rounded ends, but both are fine.

Condoms which have a mushroom top provide more sensation to the head of the penis by allowing it freedom of movement. For larger glans, these are also more comfortable.

Ribbed condoms have little nubbies on the outside which provide added sensation to the condom wearer's partner. Some like this, others find it irritating. Try switching from ribbed to unribbed if your partner has had enough extra stimulation.

Colors, Tastes And Smells

People occasionally object at first to the taste or smell of latex, but after a few experiences with condoms and enjoyable sex most people find the taste and smell of latex an erotic turn on.

Be careful about condoms which are scented as the perfume can cause allergies. There is considerable variety in the taste and smell of condom lubricants so pick what you like the best. Though most colored condoms are fine, a few have unstable dyes and run. Pastel colors are better than the real bright ones.

How Can A Person Learn To Enjoy Condoms?

• First, experiment all you want. If you're clumsy, don't sweat it. If you make a mess, open another one and start over again. If the going is easy, that's fine too.

Keep several types and sizes around so that you and/or your partner(s) will have a choice.

- Put your favorite fantasy partners into condom scenes while you masturbate. Think up ways you might get the partners to use condoms and what it would be like.

- You can't make condoms feel the exact same way as naked skin. But you can explore the sensations of latex. Once you do this, condoms often become extremely enjoyable—more like sexual enhancers than devices for sexual hygiene.

- There are a thousand ways to make putting on condoms an exciting part of sex instead of an interruption.

- Men often make the mistake of thinking that once they've put a condom on they have to ejaculate or else. This is a sure way not to enjoy condoms. Use as many condoms during sex as you like.

- Condoms cut down on friction and make some guys last longer before ejaculating. This is a wonderful feature of latex for lots of men (and women), but a problem for others. If you or your partner don't want to make sex last longer, use other low risk options until you're close to ejaculation and then put on a condom. In fact, do this as many times as you want.

- Use additional water-soluble lubricant. The lubrication on condoms helps but usually is not enough. You can heighten enjoyment by pouring just a little bit of lubricant into the reservoir tip before putting a condom on. This helps keep air out of the tip and greatly increases sensation when the lubricant seeps around the glans. It takes a little practice to get the right amount down, but is well worth the effort!

- Even the best water-soluble lubricants dry out during use. But if you wet them again, they're as good as new. So have a container of warm water around such as a squeeze bottle, sprayer, squirt gun or bowl.
- In addition to the above suggestions, ask other people who use condoms how they have learned to enjoy them the most.

How To Tell Them You Want To Use A Condom

When possible, communicate with partners about your desire to use condoms *before* you start having sex. Make it an extension of your usual sex play so that things go smoothly. Let yourself be creative! Thinking up new ways to incorporate condoms into your love life can be fun and very sexy. Talking about condoms is extremely helpful and becomes easy with practice. Be honest about your feelings. If you are nervous, embarrassed and inexperienced, say so! It gives you room to experiment and lets the other person be honest too. If you are excited by condoms, say that, too. It gives your partner a chance to explore, share tales of latex delight or deal with negative feelings, doubts and fears *before* you're in the middle of sex.

Nonverbal communication is easier or more fun for some people. You might put condoms near the place you have sex and have a copy of this book handy. Or you could simply pull one out and put it on when the right time comes around. As with other nonverbal sexual communication, it's pretty easy to tell if the other person is turned on or off. If turned on, go ahead. If turned off, you can usually smooth things over by laying the condoms aside and continuing with low risk activities.

Some people find that being very direct is the best way to approach condom use. You might say "I use condoms, how about you?" Some people love this kind of talk and others hate it. Make your approach fit your style and the occasion.

If a partner refuses to use condoms, don't fight it—do things that are low risk or let them go.

Why Condoms Don't Work and What To Do About It!

The major reason condoms fail to prevent disease is that people only use them part of the time. **Wear them every time!** Researchers state that the most common reasons people give for not wearing condoms are:

- They *think* a partner is not infected;
- They don't think condoms really work;
- They forget to carry them;
- They are too embarrassed to bring the subject up— afraid a partner will be offended; or
- They are too drunk or high on drugs to remember, care, or even be able to put their condoms on.

A CONSUMERS GUIDE TO
SOME POPULAR BRANDS AND

Shape 1: [⬭]   Shape 2: [⬭ ⟩   Shape 3: [⬭

BRAND	SHAPE	SIZE	LUBE	COLOR	TEXTURE
Trojans	1	7.5 x 2	No	Milky	Flat
Sheik Esq.	2	7.63 x 2.13	No	Clear	Slick
Kiss of Mint	2	7.63 x 2.13	No	Clear	Smooth
Lifestyles Extra Strength	2	7.5 x 2	N-9⁻	Opaque	Smooth
Lifestyles Non-lubricated	2	7.5 x 2.25	No	Opaque	Slick
Ramses Extra	2	7 x 2	N-9⁻	Clear	Slick
Mentor	3	7.25 x 2	Yes	Clear	Smooth
Mentor Plus	3	7.25 x 2	N-9⁻	Clear	Smooth
Lifestyles-Snugger Fit	3 (&5)**	6.63 x 1.88	Yes	Clear	Slick
Kimono	3 (&5)**	7.75 x 2	Yes	Clear	Smooth
Maxx	3 (&5)**	8.25 x 2.13	Yes	Clear	Smooth
Maxx Plus	3 (&5)**	8.25 x 2.13	N-9⁻	Clear	Smooth
Magnum	4	8 x 2.25	Yes	Clear	Ribbed
Excita Fiesta	4	7.63 x 2	Yes	Variety	Ribbed
Rough Riders	4	7.75 x 2	Yes	Opaque	Nubbies
Trojan Ribbed	4	7.63 x 2	Yes	Orange	Ribbed
Skin Less Skin	5	7.75 x 2	Yes	Pink	Faint bands
Crown	5	7.75 x 2	Yes	Green	Light bands
Beyond Plus	5	7.75 x 2	Yes	Green	Light bands
Saxon Ribbed	6	7.5 x 1.88	Yes	Clear	Nubs & Ribs

*Measurements are approximate due to variations in lots and difficulties in measuring. ⁻ Lubricated with Nonoxynol-9, spermicidal, anticeptic. **Shape is style 3 but sides are very slightly contoured like style 5. Copyright © 1991 Clark L. Taylor Ph.D., Ed.D. (415) 626-9511

LATEX CONDOMS
THEIR "VITAL STATISTICS"*

Shape 4: ▨▨▨▨▷   Shape 5: ▭▭▭▷   Shape 6: ▨▨▨▨▷

TASTE/SMELL	THICKNESS	OTHER REMARKS	MFG/DISTRIBUTOR
Medium/medium	Medium	the most basic	Carter Wallace
Very mild/mild	Thin	good for oral sex, light bands	Schmid Laboratories
Medium/mild	Medium-thin	very light texture, mint flavor	Ansell Inc.
Strong/medium	Thick	stronger than usual base ring	Ansell Inc.
Mild/mild	Medium-thin	extra wide, extra large at head	Ansell Inc.
Strong/medium	Thin	Lightly banded, easy to find	Schmid Laboratories
Mild/mild	Medium-thin	Adhesive inside, STAYS ON!	Mentor Corporation
Medium/mild	Medium-thin	Adhesive inside, STAYS ON!	Mentor Corporation
Medium/medium	Thin	Very lightly banded,	Ansell Laboratories
Mild/mild	Medium-thin	lightly banded, strong	Sagami/Mayer Lab.
Mild/mild	Medium-thin	lightly banded, strong, BIG	Sagami/Mayer Lab.
Strong/mild	Medium-thin	lightly banded, strong, BIG	Sagami/Mayer Lab.
Medium/mild	Very thin	Base tapers to 2″ ,strong, big	Carter Wallace
Medium/mild	Average	bright colors, medium ribbing	Schmid Laboratories
Medium/medium	Thick	Big nubbs, thick lube, strong	Ansell Laboratories
Medium/medium	Average	One of the better Trojans	Carter Wallace
Mild/mild	Ultra thin	very strong, almost no taste	Okamoto/Secure Line
Mild/mild	Ultra thin	very strong, almost no taste	Okamoto/Secure Line
Mild/mild	Ultra thin	very strong, almost no taste	Okamoto/Secure Line
Mild/mild	Medium-thin	Strongly textured, narrower	Safetex Corporation

Don't let this happen to you! If you're going to use penetration during sex, **be prepared, willing and able** to use condoms!

The second most important reason condoms don't prevent disease is they leak or break. Sometimes a condom is poorly manufactured. More often, they leak or break because they are old, have been exposed to strong sunlight, heat or extreme cold. But the most *common* reasons are rough treatment and oil-based lubricants.

Remember: *Never use oil-based lubricants on latex.* They gum up condoms, make them brittle and cause them to dissolve quickly.

If you masturbate hard during foreplay, stretch the receptacle tip or twang it on the urethra, be sure to put on a new condom before penetration, because even if the condom seems okay you may have weakened it.

If a condom breaks during intercourse, withdraw, urinate and clean up well. Partners **should not douche** as this can create small tears and spread possible infection. Consider immediately inserting a spermicide with 5% or more nonoxynol-9.

Condoms only cover the penis and therefore only protect the organ and what it touches. Unfortunately this is not enough protection against AIDS since infected body fluids which get into cuts, abrasions, ingrown hairs, pimples, bleeding gums or other broken skin may spread the disease. Be sure to check out yourself and your partner to avoid unnecessary risks. Consider putting band-aids over small problem areas as partial protection and a gentle reminder during sex. Also consider lubricants with nonoxynol-9 for problem areas not covered by a condom.

Other Latex Products

- *Diaphragms*. While the diaphragm by itself is not a complete barrier against the virus, it is an important addition to the safe sex arsenal that we are trying to have everyone develop. The first step is to make sure that the diaphragm fits correctly.

  The diaphragm which holds the nonoxynol-9 cream or jelly, blocks the cervix (the neck of the uterus that projects into the vagina). By blocking the cervix the virus is unable to gain entry into the uterus which is easily accessible to the blood supply.

- *Latex and plastic examination gloves* are superb for ass play, clitoral and vaginal stimulation, body massage and other delights. They are plain, powdered or lubricated and come in many different sizes, colors, and tastes. Gloves can be bought individually at many pharmacies and can be obtained in quantity from almost all surgical supply stores without a prescription.

- *Rubber dams* are squares of latex used by dentists to create a barrier to blood, saliva and germs during dental procedures. They are usually scented and make an excellent addition to any safe sex kit. In addition to squares, dental dam latex comes in rolls and in square yard size. Dams are available at most dental supply stores.

Lubricants and Spermicides

It cannot be said enough times—**The major reason condoms break is that they have been used with an oil-based lubricant!** Oil can be used for massage, salad dressings or lubricating automobiles but it must not be used with condoms! Unlike the rubber in tires which is hardened with sulfur to withstand heat and road conditions, the latex in condoms is "soft cured" to provide maximum elasticity and comfort. When oil is used on condoms, the latex quickly dissolves or becomes like crackly parchment.

There are many lubricants made for use with condoms. They are commonly found in pharmacies, adult book stores and grocery stores. Some popular and easy to find brands are Astroglide, Slip, K-Y Jelly, ForPlay, Ramses, Prepair and Aqua Plus.

Try out several different brands to pick the one(s) you like best. Qualities to look for are:

- How well do they lubricate?
- How long do they lubricate?
- How do they affect your skin?
- Is the lubricant in a container which prevents spills or contamination during use?
- Do you like the smell and taste or does the lubricant have positive benefits which outweigh unpleasant features?

Spermicides and Nonoxynol-9

It has long been known that the active ingredients of spermicides, primarily mild detergents, have antiseptic qualities. The most commonly used agent is nonoxynol-9. When used properly, this substance has been recognized as an important prophylactic aid against sexually transmitted diseases for over 15 years. The antiseptic nature of nonoxynol-9 was discovered when public health researchers noted that many STD-causing organisms are fragile and can be easily killed on contact with a wide variety of chemical agents. The researchers consequently set about studying common over-the-counter spermicides and "feminine hygiene" products to see if any of their ingredients would kill such pathogens. In laboratory tests, nonoxynol-9 and related detergents proved highly effective in destroying a wide variety of STDs on contact.

Nonoxynol-9 and its relatives work by bursting the outer protein cap of sperm and various disease organisms. In laboratory tests, they quickly and effectively killed herpes, gonorrhea, syphilis, CMV, yeast and trichomonas. Most recently, nonoxynol-9 also has been found to kill AIDS virus in the test tube. Pure nonoxynol-9 kills HIV outside of cells at .05% but is essentially ineffective against HIV inside of cells until it reaches a 1% concentration. Most spermicides contain between 1% and 5%. This is promising news, however nonoxynol-9 is considerably more effective under laboratory conditions than in actual sexual use because:

- The inert ingredients in spermicides—foams, gels and creams—do not always spread evenly or form a sufficient chemical barrier for nonoxynol-9 to kill pathogens before they can reach uninfected tissue.
- People often use spermicides incorrectly and only when they "think" a partner is infected.
- People abandon condoms instead of using nonoxynol-9 and condoms together.

It is very tempting to use nonoxynol-9 as a layer of prevention against AIDS while engaging in oral sex and anal intercourse, but make sure spermicides don't irritate your or your partner's genitals, mouth or rectum. When in doubt, check with your doctor. And to be sure the doctor is really up on the subject, be well informed yourself. (See "Reading Up On Condoms And Spermicides" at the end of this chapter.)

Studies show that:

1. Spermicides provide very important protection from common STD transmission if used properly and every time a person has intercourse (remember, the testing on spermicides and AIDS is incomplete). However, the effectiveness drops quickly when not used exactly as instructed on the label.
2. Spermicides and condoms used together and correctly result in much greater disease prevention effectiveness than either technique alone.
3. Nonoxynol-9 has had a very good safety record for 35

years and has been used by gays in spermicides and a couple of lubricants for anal intercourse over the last 10 years with almost no reports of problems. Animal studies of nonoxynol-9 excretion through the intestines showed no abnormalities. However, spermicides have only been tested for safe human use on the penis or in the vagina. The FDA noted in 1980 that spermicides are regularly swallowed during oral sex. Because of their extremely low toxicity and because nonoxynol-9 is used as a wetting agent in foods, the FDA deemed spermicides safe when swallowed in small quantities.

4. At this point not enough is known about the effect of nonoxynol-9 on human intestines (especially during sex) or about the AIDS virus to recommend spermicides totally without reservation for anal sex OR to recommend strongly against them! But they are certainly recommended for vaginal intercourse as a layer of AIDS prevention (provided a person is not sensitive to them—remember that changing brands usually takes care of this problem).

Research on Chemoprophylaxis

The use of nonoxynol-9 to prevent HIV/STD transmission is called "chemoprophylaxis" and the various substances which kill STDs or inhibit disease transmission are called "chemoprophylactics." Unfortunately, this is one of the most neglected areas of AIDS prevention research. There has not been a new STD chemoprophylactic introduced to the U.S. market since 1950. The development of antibiotics which easily cured STDs stunted the development of chemoprophylactics until recently when herpes and AIDS made prevention once again a burning issue.

If nonoxynol-9 were a completely effective form of prevention, the situation would not be so urgent. However, in addition to the information we have discussed above, the commercial grade of nonoxynol-9 used in most products contains impurities which are sometimes irritating and can damage cell membranes. As well, some researchers have raised the question of whether nonoxynol-9 or other mild detergents remove the mucosa from the vagina and rectum and thus leave it vulnerable to any virus not killed by common spermicides.

There are also questions about the most effective way to use nonoxynol-9 rectally. For example, to be effective, nonoxynol-9 should remain in the vagina for 4 or 5 hours after intercourse and women are advised not to douche. However, after anal intercourse, it is common to have a bowel movement. Must the nonoxynol-9 be reapplied in such cases? And how long must nonoxynol-9 remain in the bowel to be maximally effective?

In addition to the need for further research on proper use of nonoxynol-9 products for AIDS prevention, it has become apparent in recent years that the inert ingredients of "feminine hygiene" products are almost as important in forming a barrier to infection as the active ingredients. An important 1979 overview of spermicides by The

Johns Hopkins University found that the materials in the base can act as an extremely important physical barrier as well. No one has published research on the effects of various bases upon the AIDS virus.

Presently, there are a few gels with nonoxynol-9 marketed as sexual lubricants for anal intercourse. Unfortunately they have been poorly tested for effectiveness. It may be that for anal use, because of the delicate membranes and the limited mucal secretions, a different combination of inert ingredients will be required. Considerable research is being conducted on bases at the time of this printing and better products will soon be on the market.

Obviously, the amount of nonoxynol-9 required to kill HIV depends in part upon the nature of the overall product. Those products which spread well and also create a physical barrier to transmission will not need as much detergent as today's gels.

Certainly, nonoxynol-9 and its relatives are very important candidates for further research and development. However, researchers and health educators stress that there are many agents capable of killing HIV and other STDs on contact. Thus it might be that a foam, cream or gel with inert and antiseptic ingredients already approved and sold over the counter might be more effective against AIDS than any of the detergent products presently available. Some researchers feel that chemoprophylactics used in other countries should be made available in the U.S., for example products which contain chlorhexadine and benzylkonium chloride. Others insist that new, better chemical agents must be developed and tested. Unfortunately, there is little government support for such projects and the need to protect patentable discoveries and trade secrets in the private sector makes the exchange of information and rapid progress almost impossible.

A general problem in the area of chemoprophylaxis is that most research and new products are not sexologically sophisticated. Researchers ignore such factors as taste, smell and feel; yet these aspects of products seriously affect peoples' willingness to protect themselves. Also, researchers usually concentrate only on one sexual option—penovaginal intercourse. Since sexually transmitted diseases are commonly transmitted through anal sex, oral sex and injured skin as well as coitus, vaginal products are not generally designed to provide the over-all protection people need to prevent HIV/STD transmission.

The sexual lubricant industry which has grown out of the safer sex movement is an exception to this bias for contraceptive technology. Taking a sex positive perspective, many sexual lubricants aim to protect health while creating products which are sensuous, enjoyable, and appealing. Prophylactic lubricants can be applied to provide protection to a much wider area of potential STD transmission than spermicides or condoms alone. As well, though condoms and lubricants should ALWAYS be used together, we know that millions of people continue to choose protective lubricants as their first line of defense during sex. This is because lubricants are already commonly sexually acceptable for most people: they decrease friction and increase sexual pleasure.

Unfortunately, there is a wide range of product sophistication and product integrity with little guidance or support from the government or mainstream AIDS/STD researchers to improve lubricant quality. Indeed, as governmental agencies have become aware of the tremendous potential sexual lubricants present, the tendency has been to retard product development rather than encourage and support the industry. Companies which we feel deserve recognition for their continuing research and development of sensuous, effective sexual lubricants are Trimensa Corporation, Taylor-Wright Pharmacals and Techmedic-Labs. The new products these companies are bringing to market, hopefully, will protect the mucosa and reduce irritation while killing the AIDS virus and other STDs more quickly.

Sharing the Front Line of Defense

In the first edition of this book, we urged government and private industry to unite in developing AIDS/STD chemoprophylactics. We stated that the creation of a truly effective product (or combination of products) would render an invaluable service to humanity. Now we feel more strongly than ever that we must all focus intently upon chemoprophylaxic development. We must face the fact that in spite of heroic efforts, condom acceptance by the general public remains extremely low; and while we will always insist that both physical and chemical barrier protection be used in the fight against AIDS, we must invest our strongest energies into developing chemoprophylactics as a second **front line** of defense. With the advent and availability of such lubricants, we will be able to adopt a new slogan: If you do it, lube it.

Other Helpers

There are many other items which can easily create an effective barrier or kill HIV on contact. Many of these should not be placed on or in a person's body, but have a place in overall AIDS prevention.

- *Diaper wipes* often contain nonoxynol-9, alcohol and benzylkonium chloride (a substance which also kills HIV). These wipes are excellent for cleaning up during and after sex. They are great for helping take off condoms! Read the ingredients and take your choice. Some have aloe vera in them to keep skin from drying out.

- *Ordinary soaps and detergents* are very effective at killing the virus and should be used for cleaning up before and after sex.

- *Hydrogen peroxide* can be purchased from most pharmacies to be used as a gargle and for disinfecting sores or wounds. Though hydrogen peroxide comes from the bottle in a 3% solution, it kills the virus quickly even when diluted with water as low as 10 parts and can be used in many creative ways. For example it can be freshly diluted and used as an added layer of protection when rewetting water-soluble lubricants; or it can be used to sterilize latex sex toys. Leave the toys in a full strength solution for 15 minutes.

- *Ordinary rubbing alcohol* at more than 35% concentration is also very effective at killing HIV. It's not much fun in sex but is very handy to have around in case there is an emergency such as when ejaculate accidentally gets into an open sore.

- *Diluted household bleach* (1 part bleach, 10 parts water) is excellent for cleaning many sex toys and cleaning up playrooms after sex.

- *Plastic wrap* creates an effective barrier between body juices and can be a lot of fun. It shouldn't be used as a condom unless absolutely necessary. But its "see through" quality makes for a wonderful body wrap for those who need extra skin protection. It is also great to use just for the fun of it.

Reading Up On Condoms and Spermicides

There is a vast literature on condoms and spermicides. Since they are so important to AIDS prevention, here is a starter list for your further reading:

1. Department of Health and Human Services, Food and Drug Administration. "Vaginal Contraceptive Drug Products for Over the Counter Human Use; Establishment of a Monograph; Proposed Rulemaking." Federal Register, 1980 Dec. 12; pp. 82014–82049.

2. Free M., E. Skiens, M. Morrow. "Relationship Between Condom Strength and Failure During Use." Contraception, 1980 July; 22:1, pp. 31–37.

3. Hatcher, R.A. "Reasons to Recommend the Condom." Medical Aspects of Human Sexuality, 1978 August; pp. 91–92.

4. Henry, K., K. Crossley, M.A. Conant, G.Y. Minuk, C.E. Bohme, T.J. Bowen, D.I. Hoar, S. Cassol. "Condoms and the Prevention of AIDS." Journal of the American Medical Association, 1986 Sept. 19;256:11, pp. 1442–8.

5. Potts, M. and J. McDevitt "A Use-Effectiveness Trial of Spermicidally Lubricated Condoms." Contraception, 1975 June; 11:6, pp. 701–711.

6. Peter Lamptey, "Barrier contraceptives and the Interaction Between HIV and Other Sexually Transmitted Diseases" ch. 22 *Heterosexual Transmission of AIDS* Eds. N.L. Alexander, H.L. Gabelnick and J.M. Spieler Wiley-Liss: NY 1990:255–265.

7. Barbara North, "Effectiveness of Vaginal Contraceptives in Prevention of Sexually Transmitted Diseases" Ch. 23 *Heterosexual Transmission of AIDS* Eds. N.L. Alexander, H.L. Gabelnick and J.M. Spieler Wiley-Liss: NY 1990:273–290.

CHAPTER 5
Special Considerations

While the Guide is written for all people, let us take a moment to look at some of the special considerations which different populations have.

Women: Women, whether they relate to women, men, or both, have to adapt safe sex information in ways that will work with each partner. To begin this process, women need to be knowledgeable, practiced and confident about safe sex techniques. Additionally, being clear about what is sexually enjoyable is permission-giving. In the past, many women have hesitated to acknowledge this out of fear of rejection and/or abandonment but now this must change.

Many of the erotic elements and communication practices are similar for men and women. It is important to address the reality of a need for risk reduction, while being sensitive to the emotional aspects of sexual relationships. Communication between women and their partners can be clear, sweet and yet responsible. Women can be assertive, buy their own condoms, nonoxynol-9 lubricants, sponges, gloves, and dams. They can explore new ways to talk about sex by themselves, with friends, and partners.

Women grow up with many myths and constraints about sex, such as:

"Women shouldn't talk about sex." Not true. Sex is a natural function, and in the Age of AIDS, talking about sex is positive, life-affirming, hot and healthy. Talking and touching is needed in order to communicate.

"Partners and friends are uncomfortable when women talk about sex." Maybe. This is a chance that must be taken. If you talk out of genuine concern, discomfort will be lessened.

"Talking about safe sex makes me anxious." Very possibly. Practice in front of a mirror, on tape, to a trusted friend, with peers. Remind yourself that it's okay to talk about sex in general, and safe sex in particular.

"I shouldn't bring the topic up unless my partner does." Wrong. If you both wait, you take the risk of no one talking. Practice will help, successful experiences in communicating will reinforce. Sex-positive workshops, groups, counseling and therapy with nonjudgemental people can also be useful.

There are two other non-sexual concerns which must be discussed. First is the possibility of transmission through pregnancy. Both partners should be tested before pregnancy occurs. People who test positive might choose not to have children. If already pregnant, safe sex techniques with any partner are especially important. Artificial insemination should come from HIV-negative donors only. Frozen sperm is probably safer than fresh sperm.

Second is transmission during menstruation. Menstrual blood should be considered an infectious body fluid, and the uterus is more receptive to infection during menstruation. Barrier protection must be used during menstrual periods as well.

Lesbians: Lesbians have been known to have a low incidence of all STDs, so the low incidence of AIDS among lesbians is not surprising. This is probably due to the types of sexual activity lesbians participate in. An obvious reason is that semen is not involved in lesbian sex play. Semen and blood are the two most potentially dangerous body fluids. Lesbian sex does not involve semen, nor is menstrual blood likely to be transferred from one woman's vagina to the other. The implications of orally injesting menstrual blood are not known.

Nevertheless, lesbians should not consider themselves immune. We can not emphasize too often: it is not the person's identity, it is *contact* with the virus that determines the likelihood of infection. Lesbians who have sex with men, or with other women who have sex with men, should use safe sex techniques, including gloves for manual stimulation and dental dams for oral sex.

If anyone, lesbians included, engages in sex with dildos or vibrators or other sex toys, these should not be shared, nor should intravenous drug needles be shared.

Gay men: It is a tribute to the gay community's ingenuity and care, that despite the tremendous obstacles faced, they have maintained their love of life and commitment to each other. Some still do not practice safe sex and others are just beginning, but overall, the sexual changes made over the past few years are quite astounding.

There is movement from a place of sexual grief and sexual loss to one of exploration and renewed joy of sex. Developing the erotic potential of all the senses, enjoying sexual options to the fullest, exploring new ways of communicating, and creating new types of sexual relationships are priorities in the gay community. For example, those who enjoy group sex are attending J/O parties, massage parties, low-risk condom-testing parties, safe sex rituals and other events which allow them to share sensuous, erotic sexual feelings safely with other men.

Nevertheless, the work of creating gay safe sex lifestyles that are exciting, fulfilling and carefree is far from finished. The continued exploration of safe sex is needed in order to survive the present health catastrophy.

Bisexuals: We often look at the world as either "black or white," heterosexual or homosexual. The world is much more complex than that, both "grays" and bisexuals exist. In fact, the mix is not constant; as there are darker and lighter grays, there are varying interests in both the homosexual and heterosexual components. This is not to imply that bisexuality is a combination of heterosexuality and homosexuality, rather it is an entity by itself, a complete and distinct sexual orientation, where erotic attraction to both sexes is present.

Again we must emphasize the point: which sexual orientation one has, has no relationship to one's risk for AIDS. Your risk of contracting HIV is related solely to coming into contact with the virus. This means taking part in unsafe sex practices with someone who is already infected. It does not matter if these are with men or women, gay or straight or bisexual. What *does* matter is having safe sex.

There is no behavior that is bisexual. Actually, there is no behavior that is homosexual or heterosexual. What makes behavior homosexual or heterosexual is whether it is between opposite-sexed people or same-sexed people. Therefore, any behavior a bisexual engages in with a member of the same sex is homosexual and with a member of the opposite sex is heterosexual. This does not make bisexuality a less viable sexual orientation.

The media usually lumps bisexual men in with gay men when it discusses AIDS. While this is understandable to some extent, it continues the myth that these men do not have female sex partners. It is also important to note that just because a man or a woman states that s/he is homosexual, this does not mean that s/he does not have opposite sex partners.

There are many "straight" men who occasionally have sex with men—sometimes only when they're drunk or stoned, only as an experiment, only for money, or only with their best friend. A number of "gay" men periodically have sex with women—sometimes only when they're drunk or stoned, only as an experiment, only in group situations, only for money or only with their best friend. Most lesbians have sexually related to men at some point in their lives and a number still do. Some straight women are sometimes attracted to other women. Bisexual people may have desires and fantasies for both sexes, but might relate only to one or the other.

Therefore, someone's statement that they are heterosexual, homosexual or bisexual may not accurately indicate the extent of their sexual activities. Unfortunately, even before AIDS, it was unrealistic to expect complete sexual candor by prospective or even current sexual partners. Nevertheless, practicing safe sex will protect you, whether your partner is infected or not.

Swingers and group sex: Swinging is a phenomenon where people (usually couples) get together for the purpose of meeting others for sex. On-premises swing clubs, the most common type, would look to the outsider like any other party, but space is provided for the participants to engage in sex. This may be private spaces for couples, semi-private spaces for 1-2 couples, or group spaces for triads and larger groups. Off-premises clubs are usually bars, where couples meet and go back to someone's home or motel to engage in sex. There are also a variety of swinger magazines that carry personal ads which help people make contact with each other.

Swing parties are known to discourage male-male contact, though female-female contact is promoted. Drinking and drug use are minimal, since they interfere with performance. They do tend to be sexually tolerant places, so bisexual men have been known to attend. In fact, at one party house in the San Francisco area, a bisexual night was instituted for awhile (but abandoned after a few months).

The transmittability of HIV at swing clubs is not known. Preliminary studies have not shown swingers to be seropositive, but it is unknown how fast the infection would spread if the virus was introduced into the swing community. On one hand, multiple partners had been associated with the spread of HIV. On the other hand, the low level of seropositivity and AIDS among U.S. swingers is curious. Maybe the swingers have just been lucky so far. In any case, if you enjoy this behavior it can still be done using safe sex.

People whose sexual partners are in or used to be in a high risk category, including gay or bisexual men, intravenous drug users, prostitutes and their customers: You are definitely at risk. The incubation period, false negative test results, and predictable failure of resolutions to change behaviors combine to keep you at risk. It is recommended that you practice safe sex at all times.

People who used to be in a high risk category and/or have reason to believe they have been exposed to HIV: Even though you may be successful in not returning to high risk behavior, the incubation period causes you and your partner to be at risk. You may be struggling with issues such as whether or not to tell your partner, the temptation to repeat old high risk behavior, and how much faith to put in negative test results. Now is the time for total honesty between partners. You both need to discuss all the facts and make ongoing decisions about your sexual sharing.

People who are struggling with the issue of testing: This is a very complex decision which depends on many conflicting factors. Many people are so equally balanced between wanting to know and being afraid to find out that they need help in making the decision and dealing with the outcome. Don't be afraid to seek help if you are stuck. And remember, early detection of HIV infection can prolong life by making proper medical monitoring and treatment possible.

Families of adolescents: You may not know if your teenager is engaging in unsafe sexual activities or, for that matter, any sexual activity. They may not tell you if you ask. We recommend that you provide as much information as possible in any format that they are receptive to. You can also consider stocking your household with condoms and other safe sex products and encouraging their use. (Some adolescents are embarrassed to shop for these items.)

People who are in a committed sexual and/or love relationship with a partner who is seropositive or who has AIDS or ARC: This can be a most difficult situation for both parties. You will probably err in consideration of your partner and may benefit from the objectivity of a counselor and/or support group.

Families of children with AIDS or ARC: This is even more complex than a partner with AIDS and one in which professional assistance is imperative.

The worried well: While AIDS is a very serious disease, another related disease really threatens all of us. That disease has been called afrAIDS, the often irrational fear of AIDS.

It is understandable that AIDS frightens people; it is an awful disease to have. But afrAIDS has the same capacity to destroy one's life. Remember that you are much more likely to die in a car crash than you are to die of AIDS, but few of us want to ban automobiles. A rational approach to driving reassures most of us, and we are suggesting that a rational approach to AIDS will reassure the majority of those not engaging in high risk activities that they will survive this health crisis.

If knowing this, you still find you have an unreasonable or irrational fear of AIDS, join a worried well group or obtain stress reduction help from a qualified professional.

CHAPTER 6
Children, Preteens and Teenagers

When the former Surgeon General of the United States, C. Everett Koop, announced that we must embark on a massive educational campaign about AIDS that should encompass every American from the second grade up, educational planners were stunned. Immobilized by the lack of pre-existing sex education curriculum in elementary schools into which they might have inserted such instruction, they wondered out loud how to tell a seven-year-old about oral and anal sex. Parents who daily teach and caution young children about a myriad of decisions and dangers of adult life know that their question is absurd. Young children's concerns and fears about AIDS have nothing to do with their own sexual activity and cannot be allayed by a discussion of safe sex techniques.

The public hysteria about AIDS and the news and entertainment coverage of the subject make it unlikely that your child or children will not have some incomplete and perhaps disturbing idea about the phenomena of AIDS. For most young children, awareness of AIDS will fall into the vast reservoir of incompletely understood adult concerns that they don't have to worry about yet. They may never ask or may ask only cursory questions about it and show little interest if you try to engage in a lengthy discussion of the topic. The two possible exceptions are the concern some children have over the young AIDS sufferers they see on TV who have been barred from school attendance, and children who fear that their parents will "get AIDS and die," especially those who know their parents belong to a high risk group.

Although the dubious practice of scaring children into desired behavior by impressing them with dire consequences of undesired acts is a time-honored child rearing technique, it is especially destructive in the AIDS issue. Teaching young children who are still in a concrete mental process to fear sexually transmitted diseases is counterproductive to a carefree childhood and to future healthy adult sexual intimacy.

If your children are to grow up understanding the importance and anticipated joys of sexual sharing with a partner of their choice, they need you to explain and balance the possible dangers with the probable pleasures of adult sexuality. They need a continuing dialogue with a loving parent about all of the sexual issues that they may hear about and misunderstand, as well as the sexual concerns that emerge at each age and developmental stage.

The information contained in this book will provide you with the latest information on AIDS. It is up to you to determine what is appropriate and beneficial to pass on to your children and how to share the information. The important factors in this decision are:

- The age of the child.
- His/her individual characteristics.
- Your relationship with this child.
- The relevance of AIDS in the child's life.

Age

A child's age and stage of development is a critical factor in providing sexual information because children have age-specific sexual interests and concerns. The child from seven to pubescence needs to be reassured that s/he is not in danger of HIV infection or the development of AIDS or ARC. Adolescents from pubescence to sixteen need to be reassured that their sexual development will be accompanied with the desire to experience sex with another person and that this interest and desire is natural and normal. They will determine how and when their sexual sharing will occur and this decision will be based on their feelings, values, and beliefs. One of the considerations will be their knowledge of sexually transmitted diseases. Sixteen to young adults then need to know that their sexual feelings are normal and good, that their sexual choices are up to them, that the consequences of their choices are inevitable. They need to familiarize themselves with levels of risk and safe sex techniques and, if they use intravenous (IV) drugs, never to share needles.

Characteristics

The individual characteristics of your child are important and you accommodate those differences daily. AIDS education is not different. A curious, confident child can handle more information in a candid, fragmented, or offhand manner than a sensitive, brooding child who personalizes everything s/he learns.

Relationship

Your relationship is important in that some parents may not be able to speak comfortably to a child about sexual matters. Often a child will deny interest and be unresponsive to your attempts to engage in conversations about sex. They may be willing to hear it from someone else (opposite parent, sibling, teacher etc.) or they may prefer written materials or learning from overhearing your conversations with others.

Relevance

The relevance of AIDS in their lives is a critical factor. Certainly if you have a family member or close friend who is dying of AIDS your children's interest level and need to know will be dramatically increased. If you or their other parent is in a high risk category their concerns will be more personal and if, as teenagers, they enter a high risk lifestyle their need to know will be paramount.

We recommend this guide in its entirety as appropriate reading for all mid-to-late adolescents. Research indicates that the majority of young people become sexually active with a partner before they leave their teens and even if they do not, sexuality is a legitimate area of academic inquiry. Knowledge is always better than ignorance, and information about sex in general and STDs in particular will help them make better decisions about sexual activity. It is foolish, demeaning, and perhaps deadly to pretend that if they don't know about sex, they won't engage in it. It is a note of confidence from parent to adolescent to be open about the inevitability and importance of sex in our lives and to provide information and counsel about sexual issues.

We do not recommend the Guide for younger children, but rather hope that, with your new knowledge gained from it, you will feel capable and inspired to provide them information that is appropriate and timely.

How to Talk to Young Children About AIDS

Prepubescent children are not in danger of contracting AIDS. Children from seven to approximately ten or twelve need to be reassured that they are not at risk. The children who have AIDS were infected before they were born because their mother or father had AIDS (here's your chance to reinforce their knowledge about conception and gestation) or because they received a blood transfusion before doctors knew that blood needed to be sterilized. Explain that the AIDS virus is carried in the blood and that some people, who didn't even know they had AIDS, donated blood to help others. Blood transfusions are now tested and safe.

Children need to know that having AIDS does not mean you are a bad person. Reassure them that children who have AIDS are not contagious like boys and girls who have a cold, or chicken pox, or measles, because you can only get AIDS if the virus gets into your blood. They can be a friend to a child with AIDS because you don't get AIDS from casual contact, touching toys or pencils and crayons, or from coughing, sneezing etc.

They may, if they think about it, question you about receiving shots in the hospital or doctor's office. Emphasize that medical professionals use sterile disposable needles that have no germs or viruses and make sure that you enlist the nurse's support the next time they get a shot to show them that the needle is new and that it is broken and disposed of after their shot. (This is your chance to talk about the dangers of recreational intravenous drug use.) Remember, children at this age KNOW things they can see, hear, touch, taste, and smell. Germs and viruses are hard concepts to grasp.

You do not need to caution young children about sexual activity. However, they may ask you about AIDS and sex or homosexuality if they see a TV program about it or hear people discussing it. Most young children's knowledge about sex relates specifically to reproduction. What they understand and retain corresponds to their interest and curiosity about how babies are conceived and born. Although adults may be squeamish and worried about stimulating erotic interest, sexual pleasure as we know it is dependent on the hormone production of pubescence. A child's interest in sexual topics is informational/academic. Even their genital explorations are more closely related to thumbsucking, nail biting, hair twirling and blanket rubbing (which produce release of physical tension and feelings of self-nurture and security) than they are to adult eroticism.

Youngsters nearing pubescence may ask more pertinent questions about sexual activity. Since the chronological age of puberty is variable, you must be the judge of when your child is ready for more candid and detailed discussions of the sexual transmission of AIDS. As these discussions begin, the child may be overwhelmed by the complexity of it all. Many ten and eleven-year-olds vow never to have intercourse as the best method of dealing with unplanned pregnancies and sexually transmitted diseases. This is a viable choice and pronouncement for a child who has yet to experience the goal-orienting sexual focus of hormones. You need not debate the prepubescent solution of abstinence that provides a feeling of safety and security because nature will take its course and you will have many opportunities to discuss responsible sexual choices at more appropriate times. You may want to respond with an endorsement of abstinence as one solution for AIDS but suggest that it may not seem like such a good idea in a few years and that you will talk again. Some children are restrained from reopening a topic that they made an emphatic pronouncement about for fear of embarrassment and humiliation, so they need to know that you know they will change their mind later.

The germane questions about contracting AIDS by children whose parents are at risk should be answered honestly. Likewise, these same questions asked by children whose parents are not at risk can be answered honestly. Parents whose sexual life patterns and drug use patterns put them at risk need to admit, when questioned, that they are at risk, perhaps why they are willing to take that risk and how they minimize it. Children often need reassurance that their parents are not going to die.

Healthy parents who truly only have sex with each other and do not share needles can easily reassure their kids. Other parents have a more difficult situation if their children are scared. Those who have life patterns placing them in high risk may want to be tested to reassure themselves and their children that they do not have AIDS or ARC. If someone in your family has AIDS, it is a good idea to tell your children, so they can feel a part of the life and death drama that surrounds them.

Young children may also develop fears about an adolescent/young adult sibling or friend concerning high risk behavior. Siblings also often know before parents that a brother or sister is gay or bisexual. They need to know that just because someone is gay it does not mean s/he will get AIDS. Remember, as you talk about sex in general and AIDS in particular, that the child you are talking to may develop into an adult whose sexual and emotional interests are directed toward an individual of the same sex. If you are to be influential in your children's adolescent sexual choices, they must trust that they can confide their hopes, fears, feelings and dilemmas to you without fear of condemnation. If you make derogatory comments about homosexuals your child will be unable to discuss with you any same sex attractions, questions, or confusions they may experience.

Probably the most important thing to strive for is a spirit of openness within the family about sexual issues. Childhood is essentially an apprenticeship to adulthood. Children learn more about life, developing attitudes and values, *indirectly* than they do from formal instruction. By observing how you and the other adults respond to life events they develop fears or confidences about their own ability to manage life. Therefore, it is beneficial to allow children to overhear and contribute to adult conversations about important topics. They learn a lot in this casual way, but may clam up and turn off if approached directly or put on the spot.

Points to remember in talking with young children about AIDS

- Prepubescent children are not at risk.
- They can be a friend to a child with AIDS.
- Shots and blood transfusions administered by medical personnel are safe.
- Scientists and doctors are working hard to find a cure for AIDS.

- Some people will get AIDS, but most will not.
- They should never shoot drugs or share needles.
- They will have sex when they are older and they will need to know many things when that time comes in order to make good decisions about sex.
- They can ask you anything about AIDS and/or sex and if you don't know, you will find out.
- They can talk with you privately and you will respect their confidences.

We acknowledge that there is much yet to learn about AIDS, its transmission, mutations, etc. and that in reassuring children we may say things that later we find to be in error. It is important, however, that children not be tyranized by fears of possibilities over which they have no control. It makes sense to caution them about crossing streets, not playing with fire etc. but serves no purpose for them to cry themselves to sleep worrying about AIDS. We acknowledge also that there are a few prepubescent children who are drug addicted, active sexually, and/or who have been raped that may have AIDS or may have been exposed to an AIDS carrier. We have chosen not to focus on this very small segment in this volume so as to be the greatest help to the greatest number of concerned parents.

Pubescence to 15 years: How to Talk to Early Teens

Pubescence begins somewhere after the tenth year for most children. Despite the signs of inevitable maturation, children are still children at this age. Even the first years of sexual desire, potency and fertility are deemed "too early" for sex in a complex society. The early teen is interested in exploring the possibilities of relationships and bonding, but there is much to learn before they feel "ready" for sexual intercourse. Most early teens will tell you that they are just "not ready" for sex with a partner without being able to explain the parameters of readiness. Many are encouraged, goaded, seduced or challenged into sexual behavior before it is in their best interest because adults have failed to provide enough information about sexual rights, responsibilities and rewards for them to assert their right to decline, and some enter into sexual activities with peers or older partners in response to high levels of sexual interest, curiosity and desire.

The most important thing to keep in mind, as you deal with children in this age group, is that you probably will not know very much about their sexual thought and probably even less about their sexual behavior. Parents like to believe that their children would consult them first if they were in need or in trouble. However, many adolescents report that their parents would be the last to know, because they would not be able to face them. Their need to be private and self-reliant is age appropriate and a sign of strength, but it makes dealing with them about sexual matters difficult for most parents. They may try to convince you that they are not interested or that they already know everything you are trying to tell them. They may listen to what you have to say but offer nothing to sustain a dialogue for fear of revealing themselves. Your best attempts may sound like a lecture and end in frustration and anger at them for being aloof. Don't be discouraged! They still need you, but in a slightly different way. They need you to acknowledge and endorse their need to take increasing control over their own lives, but to be there in the old ways when they are overwhelmed.

Junior High School is probably the clearest demarcation between childhood and adolescence even though a group of chronological peers at this age is a study in disparity. The new school/social setting prompts even the youngest to strive for the pseudo-adult facade that is to be the hallmark of the next few years. It is when they are feeling their most mature, intellectual selves that they will agree to discuss sexual topics with adults.

Most 7th and 8th graders are more comfortable learning about sexually transmitted disease and other sexual information at school in a formal academic setting than at home, which is usually more emotional and reserved as a safe place to revert to childhood. At school, in a classroom, sex is information, data, facts you must learn. At home there is always the innuendo that if you are interested or if you ask, it is because you need to know or if parents offer, it is because they "think you're doing something." Young teens are interested and they do need to know but they want to learn dispassionately, impersonally in the abstract. They want and can handle the facts.

If your child's school has a sex education program or

is thinking of having one: get involved. Encourage it and do your best to insure that the curriculum is accurate, extensive and value-balanced with the three Rs: *Rights, Responsibilities and Rewards of Sexuality*. Everyone has a **RIGHT** to sexual expression that is not exploitive of others. Everyone, in being sexual, assumes **RESPON-SIBILITY** for the results of their sexual activity on themselves, their partner, their family and society. Everyone can enjoy the **REWARDS** of sexuality, which include physical pleasure, emotional closeness, spiritual union, procreation, relaxation, and physical and psychological health.

As a parent imparting sexual information to your teenager you may function best as a consultant. A consultant is an expert who gives information, opinion/recommendation without assuming responsibility for the ultimate decision. If the school provides the facts you can discuss the feelings and balance out the impact with family values. Young teens, when faced with the complexities and consequences of adult sexual behavior, may declare that a life of celibacy is the best way to deal with it all. It is a perfect choice for the moment and you may be tremendously relieved. But they need some indication from you that their resolve may weaken as their hormones kick into high gear and that there are joys and rewards which are unique to sexual sharing.

The government spent over 5 million dollars on "chastity education" in one year under the guise of AIDS prevention. While abstinence may seem to be a simple and effective solution it is unrealistic to believe that the majority of young people will wait more than a decade after pubescence to explore their sexuality. Surveys on teenage sexuality and developmental psychology pinpoint mid-adolescence as the time of biological and psychological readiness to begin relationships that will lead to sexual sharing. Many youngsters who have the desire and the opportunity will experiment sexually on a more casual basis in their early teens. It is more reasonable for you to accept that your adolescent will be sexual at a time that s/he will choose and that you can be influential in their decision by respecting their maturation and preparing them for adult privileges and responsibilities.

As a parent, your most important task with the early teen is to prepare your son and/or daughter to look forward to the rewards of sexual sharing despite our increasingly negative socio-sexual climate. Although you can't scare them out of being sexual you can certainly undermine the joys of sexual intimacy by instilling doubt, fear and guilt. Help your early teenager by endorsing sex as a legitimate area of academic concern, by acknowledging that sexual sharing is a healthy, pleasurable human eventuality, and by emphasizing that their sexual choices will have a significant impact (good or bad) on their own lives, the lives of others and society at large. Provide age appropriate books on human sexuality including materials on the history of sex, the politics of sex, sex and religion, sexual art, sexual health etc. Before antibiotics, other venereal diseases were incurable and epidemic. Junior high school students like to contemplate and discuss the similarities and differences of topics that interest them. They like to be in the know.

Discuss the topic of AIDS with your spouse/partner/adult friend casually in your household as you hear about it on radio or TV or read about it in magazines and newspapers. Let your teenagers overhear and contribute to these conversations as they wish. Give them recognition for their knowledge on the subject. Ask them if kids their age worry about getting AIDS (most do not, because they do not see themselves at risk). *Do not try to scare them into a personalized fear of an AIDS death*. If they have developed a personal fear of AIDS, reassure them with proper precautions, i.e. no drug use ever and safe sex techniques when it's time to be sexual so they need not fear contracting AIDS.

Points to remember in talking to early teens about AIDS:

1. Don't try to scare them into a personalized fear of AIDS.
2. See that they have access to the facts.
3. Know the curriculum of the sex education class at school.
4. Encourage their participation in and contributions to family conversations about AIDS.
5. Respect their maturation and help them consider their sexuality a wonderful part of their total being. Know that they will be sexually active when they feel ready.

129

6. Keep talking even if they don't talk back. Discuss new findings and your thoughts and feelings about them but don't put them on the spot.

7. Remember the Rights and Rewards of sexuality each time you talk about the Responsibilities of sex.

8. Know that this is the age of value formations and that they are interested in the history, politics, and ethics of sexuality as well as the practical aspects of sexual activity.

9. Review the points to remember for younger children and incorporate those that are still applicable for your child.

10. If you have reason to believe your teen is sexually active, review the next section and consider letting them read all or parts of this Guide.

Late Teens From 16–20 Years
How to Talk to Late Teens

Adults have always been reluctant to provide sexual information to teens. They have many reasons which all basically mean they are afraid that if teens know about sex they will be sexual. Actually, young people have sex when they decide they are "ready." Now adults have an even greater fear that you will have sex and/or use drugs and get AIDS. Because they don't want you to die (and because they know you will be sexual sooner or later), adults are becoming more willing to provide information about sex and sexually transmitted diseases.

Even the Surgeon Generals of the United States make

public declarations that we must educate everyone about AIDS. Tell adolescents that it is very important that they know all that there is to know about AIDS so that when they decide to be sexual with a partner they can have sex responsibly and safely.

As adults you have grown up in a time that has provided effective birth control methods, legal abortions and successful treatment of venereal diseases. It has been pretty tempting to be nonchalant and even irresponsible about sexuality. Although the negative consequences of irresponsible sex were pretty scary at the time, you could get through it. Many young people learned some lessons about sex the hard way through trial and error, but they survived. When the consequence is AIDS, you don't survive. AIDS is fatal. There is no cure and there is no immunization against the AIDS virus.

If you are a teen and reading this, remember it's often hard to take adult warnings seriously in your teens because you feel invincible. However, the risks are real and you need to make some important decisions about sex and drugs. There is a lot that we don't know about AIDS, but the things we do know can save your life.

The danger of AIDS is especially problematic for teens for many reasons.

- Sexual interest, curiosity and desire are high teenage priorities.
- Even though you may be scared about AIDS, your natural, normal, healthy, biological sexual drive is strong and demanding.

- Most teens have few or no resources of accurate information about sexual matters and counsel.
- Teens are reluctant to talk to any adult about their sexual activity.
- Sexual experimentation with more than one partner is common in mid to late teens.
- Many teens are also experimenting with drugs.
- Spontaneous, opportunistic sexual encounters may find you unprepared to protect yourself from pregnancy and STDs.
- Inexperience, lack of knowledge and embarrassment make it difficult to negotiate for safe sex practices.
- Teens (especially girls) are reluctant to buy, carry and use condoms.
- Many girls use no protection at all against pregnancy or STDs.
- Many girls have sex for nonsexual reasons and do whatever the boy wants because they want the boy.
- Girls who have sex with older men might choose partners who are in high risk groups.
- Girls might have sex with boys who are having sex with other boys/men or prostitutes.
- Boys might have sex with other boys/men or prostitutes.
- Homosexual or bisexual boys might have high risk sexual activity with partners in high risk groups.

We recommend that all sexually active teenagers read and reread this Guide, share it with friends and refer to it often. Find a knowledgeable adult with whom you can discuss your personal sexual concerns—someone you trust enough to tell everything. If you have done something sexual you think may have placed you at risk, tell that person so they can help you put it in perspective, do the appropriate thing, and stop worrying.

If you need personal information and wish to remain anonymous, call a sex information hotline. If there is no sex information hotline in your area try the emergency telephone services that are available. Many health professionals will talk with you if you call and say "I'm 16 years old and I need to talk to someone about AIDS."

Professionals You Might Call:

- Sex therapists are usually not listed separately in the yellow pages. You will find them under the headings of Psychologists, Marriage, Family and Child counselors, Clinical Social Workers. If they specialize in sex counseling it will be noted under their name.
- Medical doctors are listed twice in the yellow pages under Physicians, alphabetically and by speciality. The doctors who should know the most about AIDS are: a) Infectious disease specialists. b) Urologists—who diagnose and treat disorders of male genitalia and male and female urinary problems. c) Gynecologists—who diagnose and treat disorders of female genitalia and reproductive organs.
- Community services.
  - AIDS Foundation Hotlines. Large cities have many services for people who have AIDS or fear they have been exposed to AIDS.

- The gay community may also have a variety of services including support groups to help their members deal with personal fears and crisis.
- STD clinics are a service of city or county health services which provide information, testing, diagnosis, and treatment.
- AIDS antibody testing is available through private physicians or public clinics. Please review Chapter 2 of this Guide if you are contemplating being tested.

As you study this Guide you will learn a lot about AIDS that will help you understand the sexual implications. In order to know what to do about it you must:

- Determine your level of risk.
- Take responsibility for yourself.
- Practice safe sex.

How to Determine Your Level of Risk

Understand that HIV is transmitted sexually by exchanging body fluids with an infected partner. It is also transmitted by sharing intravenous drug needles with an infected person.

Know that it is highly unlikely that you will know if your partner has been exposed to the virus. They might not even know.

Know that if you are a homosexual or bisexual boy, you might engage in high risk sex acts with partners who are in a high risk category. Use safe sex techniques every time you have sex with anyone.

Know that the more sexual partners you have, the greater possibility you have of exposure to AIDS and other STDs.

Know that if you have unsafe sex you increase your risk of exposure.

How to Take Responsibility for Yourself

Understand that if you get it, you've got it, and it doesn't make any difference who gave it to you or how sorry you are.

Know that no one cares as much about your life and health as you do.
Don't think that you can fool yourself and sneak around these principles. You may luck out, but then again you may not.

How to Practice Safer Sex

Know that barriers which prevent the exchange of body fluids are your best line of defense and that the use of spermicides make them even safer.

Buy and *use* condoms lubricated with nonoxynol-9. Sexually active boys and girls should carry condoms.

Know that you can purchase condoms in any drug store, no questions asked.

Know that boys can also be infected by girls and that condom use protects you both.

Know that if you give a boy the choice of sex with a condom and no sex without a condom, he will choose sex. (The choice should *never* be sex with or without a condom.)

Don't have sex when drunk or high. Sex is its own high.

Don't share needles and don't have unprotected penetration sex with anyone who does or has in the past shared needles.

Know that the desire, urgency and pleasure of the moment are not worth the risk of unprotected sexual intercourse.
Don't be talked into unprotected sex because neither of you have condoms or because the boy says it isn't natural, doesn't feel as good, he won't love you anymore, he'll find someone else or any other excuse.

Don't be talked into sex for nonsexual reasons. Don't believe that if you give sex because your partner wants it, s/he will like you better or longer. They might just like sex and be willing to say anything to convince you to have it.

Don't depend on your partner to provide protection or good judgment in all sexual situations. S/he may put pressure on you when drunk or high or particularly horny. You need the courage to stand firm even if you are begged or threatened.

Know that many young people reserve sexual intercourse for marriage or a committed relationship.

Know that most of the sexual activities called petting, including mutual masturbation to climax, are safe (and satisfying).

You have the right to be sexual and to know everything you want or need to know about sex. The consequences of sex can change your life and you accept the responsibilities when you decide to engage in sex. The rewards of sex enhance the quality of life and are enhanced when you make responsible decisions and choices. Remember the three R's of sex: Rights, Responsibilities and Rewards.

CHAPTER 7
How to Create
A Safer Sex Lifestyle

The right way to create a safer sex lifestyle is the
way that works for each of us. The suggestions
and exercises in this chapter are simply a guide to
help you along the way. They are based upon strategies
developed over the past years of giving safe sex workshops. These are the best techniques we know to help
people reduce risk, improve their sex lives and reclaim
the joy of sex.

We begin with safer sex activities and exercises that
can be done alone for personal sexual growth and
change. Then we explore interaction with other people—
mates, lovers, dates, and friends. You may wish to try
out this sequence for yourself or you may prefer to skip
around, picking activities and exercises which seem
more important to work on first—it's *your* sex life and
it's all up to you! In making your decisions you might
wish to take the following observations into consideration.

We have learned from ourselves and others that when
we expand our personal sexual base we are often happier
and more able to create and maintain the kind of sexual

relations we enjoy. Exploring our personal sexual feelings, desires, sensuality and eroticism is therefore both a gift to ourselves and to those we love.

Our whole body, from the top of our heads to the soles of our feet, is a virtual banquet of potential sensual, erotic, orgasmic delights. Most of us view our possible sensual and sexual outlets from the perspective of an impoverished menu. That is only a negative illusion. There are, in fact, an abundance of options available to all of us and the limitations created by AIDS need not diminish that abundance. If embraced, the concepts here awaken us to a rich way of dealing with our sexuality so that, even after AIDS has been conquered, our way of relating to ourselves and others will have been improved greatly. This is the concept which guides each section of this chapter.

Reclaiming Our Personal Sexuality

Reclaiming our personal sexuality is a great, absolutely safe way to begin recovering the other parts of health and psychological well-being that have been affected by AIDS. It also reduces the AIDS sexual trauma and fear which sometimes causes people to stop taking good care of themselves.

It is possible to regain the spontaneity and much of the freedom that existed before AIDS by practicing safe sex techniques until they become automatic. People mourning the loss of spontaneity which results from needing to think and act carefully at first, should remember this fact. It is also good to remember that while we think we are spontaneous, many of us are in a rut. Many people have sex at the same time of day or night, using the same activities, taking the same positions, making the same sounds, and using the same sexual toys and products. Thus, instead of feeling a loss of spontaneity many of us are experiencing loss of familiar behavior and reluctance to changing familiar patterns.

In our practices and workshops we come across many people who have overcome such initial reactions, made significant changes in their sex lives and are once more enjoying their sexuality. Many report their lifestyles are much more satisfying than before the Age of AIDS. There is a central theme which runs through the experience of such people:

When we view safer sex as an opportunity to explore and play, to be truly spontaneous, it becomes an adventure—one which continues to bring new zest and thrill to our love lives.

Although we have developed a sequential process, give yourself permission to begin wherever you feel most appropriate for your needs. For example, some of us need to reduce high risk sex with others before we can work on an overall program. This is particularly true of those who are just becoming aware of the sexual aspects of AIDS transmission and are accustomed to having high risk sex with many partners. In this situation, the most productive approach is often to start with the highest risk activities first. Such an approach can prepare the way for exploring self sexuality later—learning how to increase orgasmic potential and sexual enjoyment and meeting sexual needs with the lowest risk activities.

Now that we've covered the basics of the present chapter, let's get set, ready and GO!

Getting Started

Start with a *willingness* to acknowledge that:

- Our sexuality is an integral part of who we are.
- It is good for our bodies to give and take pleasure.
- We are the only ones who can reclaim our sexuality—no one else can do it for us.

Take Time For Yourself

A good way to begin developing your personal safer sex lifestyle is to create a special time and safe space for yourself to explore the suggestions and exercises contained in this chapter. About an hour a day is optimal. Find an hour that will fit comfortably into your schedule and lifestyle and claim it for your personal sexual growth. These suggestions may help:

- Have a frank discussion with yourself, your partner, your children or any housemates about respecting the hour you take for yourself. Be firm. *"Don't bother me unless it's a real emergency. This is my private time!"*
- Put a "Do Not Disturb" sign on the bedroom door and lock it.

- Take a realistic look at your daily activities so you can evaluate priorities in taking time for yourself.
- Reschedule your duties and appointments so you have no distractions or temptation to skip your adventure.
- Schedule a regular hour each day for your explorations.
- Make a place in your home (or wherever you spend the most time) that is sexy, sensual, soft, and quiet.
- Explore and discover books, pictures, music, textures, and/or smells that are especially sensuous, enjoyable, erotic and arousing to you and be willing to add them to your environment.

My special time each day is going to be:

_____

_____

_____

My special place is going to be:

_____

Things I'm going to add to my environment are going to be:

_____

_____

_____

Prepare for a good time now! Go shopping and buy something new for your safer sex lifestyle. For example, it could be something for massage or bathing, a piece of sensuous clothing, a big pillow, a new type of condom or lubricant, a vibrator or a new dildo. See how inexpensive and creative you can be. Dime stores, drug stores, toy shops, hardware stores and secondhand places can provide amazing safer sex toys!

Make A Personal Contract For Changes In Your Sexual Lifestyle

Under the best of conditions it takes courage and commitment to learn new ways of relating sexually. The problems and feelings which sexual change ordinarily bring up are compounded by the pressure of AIDS and the social atmosphere of repression and confusion in which we live.

One way to help change our sexuality toward risk reduction and personal enrichment is to make a contract. The more willing and agreeable we are to do some exploring for and of ourselves, the more growth we are likely to experience. And though it takes courage to get started, most people find that many changes are delightfully easy to make and immediately gratifying, while others take time and effort.

In the space provided here, define for yourself what you are committed to working on. If you have a cooperative partner, list what you are willing to work on together. What are some of your worries about making a commitment to change? What will be scary about making the current situation "better" or "different"? List some aspects of your sexlife you should not change at all and say why they should stay the same.

- Start with the easiest and least threatening changes to make in your contract and build from there.
- Remember that change does not happen overnight. While a slip backwards into risky sex can be dangerous, it is not an excuse to discontinue your commitment to change.

My Personal Contract For A Hot and Healthy Safer Sex Lifestyle

_____

_____

_____

_____

_____

_____

_____

_____

Make Your Contract A Living, Changing Agreement

As you go about exploring your decisions, you may find that some are not as important as others, that some changes which seemed desirable don't work out, and that other options come up that are better than anything you wrote into your original contract. To take these possibilities into account, make your contract a living, changing agreement. Refer to it often and keep updating it as you go along.

This Is How I'm Going To Make My Safer Sex Lifestyle Even Better!

_____

_____

_____

_____

_____

_____

_____

_____

Empowering Your Contract

Whatever changes you decide to make, putting them into practice is what counts. Some ways to internalize and actualize these changes might be:

- **_Create Affirmations_** and say them out loud in front of a mirror. For example, "I can create these changes. They will be enjoyable. I can get personal support, cooperation and enthusiasm from my partner(s)."
- **_Create Visualizations:_** After a peaceful and relaxing meditation, keep your eyes closed and, with as much detail as possible, imagine yourself creating the changes you want and need to make. See your life unfolding with as much joy, pleasure, safety and sensuality as you want.

- *Tie a string around your finger* or better yet, place brightly colored objects around your environment. Each time you notice one, take a deep breath and remind yourself that you can make the changes you need to make and also keep your sexuality alive and vital. You may want to choose or buy something to wear that will serve the same purpose.

- *Find a support person or group* that you can talk with on a regular basis. Report progress you've made, process feelings that arise, work through resistance, get ideas, and know that you are not alone in your concerns. Your support person may be your spouse, lover, a sexual partner, friend or relative. But whomever you choose, it is most important that they be *nonjudgmental* and *supportive* and that you feel some degree of rapport and trust with them. If you join a group, it may be an informal group of friends, a women's group, worried well group, a church group or a more formalized group with counselors or facilitators. Again, you should feel a sense of trust, rapport and confidentiality.

Keep a Journal and/or Scrapbook

Journals are great for keeping track of progress and checking in on how we feel. Journals can be like diaries or outrageous creations—a box full of jotted down thoughts, mementos of safe sex experiences, safe sex stories and pictures, photos of you and your new safer sex friends—whatever you want.

It's useful to keep a safe sex scrapbook as well. Here you can paste in the latest information on AIDS transmission and prevention. If you collect a lot of materials you may prefer to have a special file box. One person we know pasted sexy safe sex pictures all over her file box so it was more thrilling to work on.

Create a Schedule of Activities

One of the most effective ways to achieve your safer sex lifestyle goals could be to decide on a definite period of time for intense work—six weeks, two months, a month. Then create a plan of action. Put it down on paper! Do it your own way.

This is an example to help you start thinking about a plan:

WEEK 1—This week I'm going to work on being my own best sexual partner!!!

Monday—During my special safer sex hour, I'll take a bubble bath with music and incense. Maybe I'll put a mirror near the tub, so I can see myself bathe. Then after my bath, I'll give myself a massage with a new special lotion.

Tuesday—I'll start doing those breathing and Kegel exercises to increase the control and power of my orgasms. I'll also massage myself with a vibrator, an ostrich feather, a silk scarf and something furry. I'll let myself moan and groan as much and as loud as I want.

Wednesday—I'll continue those exercises and map my body to find erogenous zones I might not know I have. Am I still a virgin anywhere? I think I'll also try creative masturbation. Maybe the things I used for massage yesterday will come in handy. Maybe I'll add a few things or maybe I'll see just how long I can last or what it feels like to keep getting close to orgasm but stopping.

Thursday—I'll do my exercises, then I'll massage myself in new places (maybe the inside of my nose, my mouth, my ears and my asshole). Then I'll practice masturbating in lots of new, different positions.

Friday—I'll put it all together. I'll take a new type of creative bath and massage myself all over, wet and in the tub, then with the towel and then with everything else in sight. Then, I'll put the mirror in a room I've never used before and I'll really go to town having fun. I'll try out total body masturbation, multiple orgasms. Maybe I'll even try out putting on a sexy costume. I wonder what it would be like wearing a mask and masturbating in front of the mirror?

Saturday—I'll spend my special time reflecting on the week and meditating on my sexuality. Then I think

I'll review my contract and see if there's anything I'd like to change. I'll also write in my journal and bring my AIDS prevention scrapbook up to date.

Sunday—I'll plan next week. I want to work on dating skills and creating a safe space for touch.

Again the schedule above is just an example. Make the schedule fit your own individual personality, special needs and growth objectives!

Breathing, Sensory Awareness and Sexuality

Breathing, like sexual response, is a naturally occurring event in the body; however, awareness and control of the rate and rhythm of our breath is not. Learning to become aware and in control of our breathing is a powerful tool in learning to relax, reducing stress and anxiety, helping our bodies to function at an optimal level, and for prolonging, increasing and maintaining sexual pleasure and health!

We find that it is very useful to incorporate breathing exercises into the process of creating a safe sex lifestyle at a very early stage. The exercises which help us relax make it easier to explore the more charged sexual subjects, while the ones which increase sexual vigor and enjoyments help create greater interest in the overall process of sexual change.

We also concentrate on sensory awareness here at the beginning of "How To Create A Safer Sex Lifestyle" because people often equate sex with genital feelings only and are out of touch with the many enjoyable, often intensely sexual pleasures that other parts of the body can give. To make safer sex more enjoyable, more powerful, more satisfying sex, let's really get into using all our senses!

Breathing

Usually, we only take in a small portion of the air our lungs are capable of containing. Taking a really deep, complete breath helps purify and oxygenate our blood. It also focuses our attention on the "here and now," so that our minds don't run away with the fear and anxiety of negative fantasies. It is natural and more powerful to expand our bodies as we inhale and to contract our bodies as we exhale.

Abdominal Breathing

The purpose of this exercise is to develop comfortable and relaxed breathing in the pelvic region. (This is called abdominal or diaphragmatic breathing.)

Begin by lying on the floor or a bed with arms at your side and legs uncrossed. A small pillow under the head or neck might make you more comfortable. .Close your eyes and begin breathing slowly, inhaling through the nose and exhaling through the mouth.

Now place one hand lightly on your lower abdomen. Concentrate on the movement of your abdomen as you breathe. Push your hand upwards with your abdomen as you inhale, letting the abdomen fall as you exhale. Now, breath in slowly, and as you exhale, use your hand to push your breath out further than you normally do. Imagine the air slowly filling your abdomen and emptying with a woosh or sigh. Exhale at the same rate as you inhale.

Make sure you exhale more fully than you normally do. Pause after each exhalation and don't rush. Do this ten times. How often do you allow your belly to stick out?

Synchronous Breathing

This exercise is designed to harmonize your breathing and heart rate. Many people find that coordinating these two important rhythms brings an increased sense of well-being.

As you inhale, count the beats of your pulse; this is your breathing number. Write it down right here _____ . The number may change. Use this one for the exercises in breathing.

Inhale to your number.
Hold for one-half your number.
Exhale to your number.
Hold for one-half your number.

As you develop a feeling for this synchronous breathing technique, your body sensations and your breathing rate will begin to change and harmonize with your pulse rate. Continue breathing in this way for three minutes each time or until you feel your heart pulse and breathing have stabilized and synchronized. Do not work for more than 10 minutes total to start with.

Genital Focus Breathing

Breathe in through your nose and then imagine that you are breathing out through a four inch diameter pipe in your genitals! Exhale through your crotch. Repeat this six times, eyes closed.

Complete Breath

1. Stand easily and erectly with arms at sides. Exhale through your nose; empty the lungs completely.
2. Slowly inhale through the nose to a count of nine. As you inhale first push out your abdomen and then your entire chest.
3. While inhaling slowly bring your arms overhead and simultaneously rise on toes. Count nine to complete movements 2 and 3. Touch palms overhead at count of nine. Hold for a moment.
4. Slowly exhale through your nose to a count of nine; as you exhale, lower your arms slowly and return heels to floor.
5. Repeat without pause, 4 to 10 times.

Chest Expansion

1. Stand easily and erectly; slowly raise arms to shoulder level. Bend elbows, bringing hands in to touch chest, palms outward.
2. Move arms out and straighten back as far as possible without strain. Clasp hands behind back and straighten arms. Count five for each of these movements.
3. Gently bend backward from waist as far as possible without strain. Hold.
4. Bring clasped hands, arms straight, up over back and bend forward as far as possible. Relax neck and hold.
5. Slowly straighten up. Unclasp hands. Relax.

Pelvic Breathing

The purpose of this breathing exercise is to coordinate pelvic movement with breathing.

Lie down on your back on the floor or bed with arms at your sides and legs uncrossed. Breathe slowly, using abdominal breathing for a few minutes to establish your rhythm. Close your eyes. As you inhale, press your bottom toward the floor and let the air fill your abdomen. As you exhale, imagine that your pubic bone is being magnetically drawn towards the ceiling. The magnet is attached right to the clitoris or penis. Your pelvis will slowly tilt up as you exhale. Repeat this at least ten times. It is important to have the pelvis tilt backwards on the inhalation and tilt forward on the exhalation. The abdomen continues to fill out as you push your bottom down towards the floor.

Do the same exercise while kneeling with your hands flat on the floor in front of you. As you inhale, push your bottom towards the ceiling and let your belly hang down low at the same time. Arms are still. As you exhale, push your pelvic bone towards the floor, forward. Repeat this six times.

Rag Doll

1. Stand with feet apart. The distance of one foot from the other should approximate the distance from shoulder to shoulder.
2. Lean forward from the waist, allowing your arms, neck and head to dangle from your trunk. Don't force your fingertips closer to the floor. Allow the upper portion of your body to go limp. Next, slowly return to an erect posture starting from the lower back and moving upward until you are in the beginning position. Repeat three to five times.

Pelvic Tension Breaker

1. Stand easily and erectly; place your fists just below your waist in back; place feet apart at shoulder distance from each other with toes pointing inward.
2. Slowly arch your back; press fists into pelvis using as much pressure as possible; allow head and neck to fall backward.

3. Rock back and forth between heels and toes, increasing pressure of fists with each movement and maximum amount of pressure is being exerted on your pelvis.
4. Return feet to position flat on floor. Hold to count of five.
5. Slowly return to standing. Relax. Repeat three to five times.

Kegel Exercises

These exercises are designed to strengthen and give you voluntary control over a muscle called the pubococcygeus muscle (pew-bo-kak-se-gee-us), or P.C. for short. This muscle is the support muscle for the genitals in both men and women. There is a definite correlation between good tone in the P.C. muscle and orgasmic intensity.

These exercises can help you to:

1. Increase your awareness of feelings in your genital area.
2. Increase blood circulation in the genital area.
3. Add to your sexual responsiveness.
4. Aid in restoring vaginal muscle tone following childbirth.
5. Increase your control over your orgasm.

To find your P.C. muscle, when you need to urinate, see if you can start and stop the flow of urine with your legs apart (without moving your legs together). The P.C. muscle is the one that stops the flow. If you don't find it the first time, don't give up; try again the next time you need to urinate. Men can sit or stand.

Slow Kegels
Tighten the P.C. muscle and hold it as you did when you stopped the flow of urine for a slow count of 3. Then relax the muscle.

Quick Kegels
Tighten and relax the P.C. muscle as rapidly as you can. At first it will feel like a flutter. You will gradually gain more control.

Pull In/Push Out
Pull up the entire pelvic area as though trying to suck up water into the genitals. Then push out or bear down as if trying to push the imaginary water out. (This exercise will use a number of "stomach" or "abdominal" muscles as well as the P.C. muscle.)

Repetitions: At first do ten of these exercises (one set), 3 times a day (3 exercises × 10 × 3 times a day = 90 total exercises to start). Each week add 5 more times to each exercise. Example: Week 2—3 sets × 15 times × 3 times a day; Week 3—3 sets × 20 times × 3 times a day; Week 4—3 sets × 25 times × 3 times a day. Keep doing 3 sets a day.

You can help yourself remember to do the exercises by associating them with some activity you do every day: talking on the phone, watching television, waiting in line, or lying in bed. Think of activities which don't require much moving around.

Don't worry if your muscles seem to get tired easily at first; that's normal for exercising any new muscle group. Rest between sets for a few seconds and start again. Remember to keep breathing naturally.

Women can place one or two fingers into the vagina and men one finger on each side of the base of the penis in order to feel the movement and strength of the muscle. You may also watch the movement by looking at your genitals in a hand mirror. Doing these things with your Kegels will help you learn them more rapidly.

Sensuous Bathing

Bathing is an excellent way to increase personal sensory awareness and discover new erotic sensations. We recommend that you first try this process by yourself and then with your spouse, lover, partner, or friend.

Simple Pleasures

Take a sensuous bath or shower not just to get clean but to experience touching and exploring your body with your hands—nurturing yourself. In addition to your hands, you might explore the sensations of such items as sponges, complexion brushes, plastic pompoms, or anything your heart desires. Treat yourself royally! After you dry off, lie down in a quiet place and reflect on the experience.

An extraordinary bathing experience

Plan an absolutely extraordinary bathing experience for yourself. Get relaxed and think about what would be really luxurious and unusual. To assist in this process, we have made a few suggestions. Pick and choose as you like and, of course, add anything else you want!

- Visit a store or shopping center that has a bathroom boutique or skin care center.
- Smell the bath oils, crystals, soaps and scents.
- Feel the loofas, sponges, foot and scalp massagers.
- Get ideas on how you can make your bathing experience more sensuous.
- Treat yourself to something luxurious. It does not have to cost a great deal. The important thing is that it makes you feel good.
- Establish a time when you can have your bathroom all to yourself for at least an hour.
- Create the environment so it fits your delight as much as possible. That may mean adding music, candles, incense, bubble bath, fresh clean towels, or anything else you can think of, to your bathroom.
- Draw as hot a bath as feels comfortable and, while you are waiting for it to fill, relax and do nothing.
- Add your favorite oils, crystals, or scents to the water and invite yourself into the tub.
- Lay back and just relax. Let the water flow over you. Breath, fantasize, listen to the music and let go of all the concerns of the day. This is for you. Breath and enjoy.
- Slowly begin caressing your body with the hot, slippery, wet water. Slower still, begin running your finger tips over your face. Feel every part of your face, eyelids, cheeks, nose, nostrils, ears, etc.

- Explore your entire body. Don't forget the parts of your body you avoid. Start anywhere you please.
- If you start with your scalp, you might:
  - completely soak your head
  - firmly and slowly run your fingers through your hair and over your scalp
  - briskly massage your entire head with your fingertips
  - take a hand full of hair, pull hard and hold for the count of ten
  - let go and notice the tingling
  - repeat this so your entire scalp is alive
  - now, gently stroke your hair and be aware of the difference
  - soak your head again and take time to appreciate and enjoy.
- Move to another part of your body—your arm, breast, nipple, thigh, foot, ass, etc. We are going to do a similar kind of sensate focusing here:
  - lovingly caress that part of your body that you have chosen to play with just now
  - begin to tap that area
  - take a soapy sponge or loofa and brush
  - increase the pace and pressure
  - stop and notice the tingling sensation
  - gently pinch the same area
  - let go and pinch again—harder
  - let go and, as hard as you can without hurting yourself, firmly pinch and hold until the count of ten

- let go, just barely pat and become aware of the aliveness
- continue focusing in the same area at your own pace.
- Experiment in the same way with the rest of your body. Give extra time to the parts you rarely touch or rarely touch sensuously:
  - when you have finished notice how alive your entire body feels
  - take a few moments to reflect and completely enjoy the experience
  - lovingly pat yourself dry
  - luxuriate as you slowly apply body cream, lotion, oil or talc
  - look in the mirror, feel good and thank yourself.

Bathing with a partner

Let's jump ahead for a moment to partnered experiences. When you are ready to exchange this bathing experience with someone else, choose a person you care a great deal about. Keep in mind that neither you nor your partner have to do anything that feels uncomfortable. However, don't use this as an excuse not to really and lovingly extend your limits. Remember orgasms are not the focus of this section. If they should happen, fine, but don't go looking for them. Teach your partner some of the things you have discovered and try looking at them as a completely new person. As you bathe your partner let each step of the process teach you something new about them. When it is your turn to be bathed, give yourself permission to totally let go, relax and be taken care of.

A few tips that can make bathing together more adventurous and enjoyable

- Before your partner arrives, remove from sight everything possible that says "This is a bathroom"—toothpaste, medicines, douche bags, clothes hampers.
- Redecorate to create an unusual environment. Use flowers, unusual drape cloths (satin, velvet, synthetic leopard skin, whatever would turn you both on).
- You will have more room and enhance the atmosphere if you take down the shower curtain or remove the sliding doors from a tub.
- You can most easily bathe a partner's feet and lower legs if you sit on the edge of the tub. Be sure to place a towel where you sit to avoid the cold tub and to soften the sliding door metal guides.
- A large sea shell or unusual wooden or plastic container can be wonderful for pouring water over your partner and self.
- Candles and music do wonders for transforming a bath into a magical experience.
- One way to bathe your partner's upper body is to sit behind your partner so that his/her back rests upon your chest. Then reach around his/her body to wash and explore. This can be a very nurturing experience.
- Have several ways planned to end the bath so that you have pleasant alternatives from which to choose—a nap, a massage, a light meal.

Safer Sex Fantasies

Fantasies are a powerful tool in:

- Creating a safer sex lifestyle;
- Defining and clarifying your feelings;
- Enriching your sexual experiences, either alone or with a partner; and
- Enhancing intimacy and trust with a partner when the fantasies are shared.

While most of us fantasize frequently, we don't have the time, energy, ability or the desire to act out most of what we fantasize about. Many people forget that fantasy is not reality and feel guilty if their sexual fantasies are nontraditional, politically incorrect or otherwise "inappropriate." *Nobody will ever get AIDS from a fantasy* even if the activities in the fantasy are unsafe.

While fantasies can't force us to do things we don't want to do, we can use fantasies to empower action. Therefore, it is extremely important to create and explore fantasies. Here are some exercises that will help.

The Safer Sex Fantasies Multiple Choice Lottery. Pick as many as you want—*Everybody can win! I feel sexual fantasies are:*

_____ a great way to get turned on

_____ immature

_____ boring

_____ something I can do and still be celibate

_____ fun to verbalize

_____ my own business

_____ the same as behavior

_____ sinful

_____ enriching to my sex life

_____ wrong if they involve thoughts of violence

_____ fun to share with the right partner

_____ sometimes politically incorrect

_____ safe

_____ something my parents never did

_____ a hindrance to the full enjoyment of sex

_____ innocent

_____ wrong while having sex with a partner

_____ fun to act out

_____ dangerous if about unsafe sex practices

_____ something everyone does

_____ orgasmically oriented

Safer sex fantasies are something I can have while . . .

_____ talking on the phone

_____ reading a letter from mom

_____ petting the cat

_____ talking to a friend with AIDS or ARC

_____ grocery shopping

_____ working in the garden

_____ making love

_____ looking at porno

_____ eating lunch
_____ sleeping
_____ taking a shower
_____ reading this book
_____ learning about AIDS
_____ creating a safer sex lifestyle
_____ in the bathroom
and _____ , _____ , _____

Fantasies . . . OH, Ahhh, ahhh

_____ I like to fantasize (daydream) about sex
_____ when alone, _____ when with a partner,
_____ When I'm with a group of people.
_____ There's only one kind of fantasy that turns me
on.
_____ I like to experiment with different kinds of
fantasies.
_____ I like to share my fantasies _____ with lots of
other people, _____ my partner.
_____ I like to act my fantasies out

If I were to act out my sexual fantasies I'd be:

_____ happy
_____ very happy
_____ exhausted
_____ disappointed
_____ embarrassed
_____ breaking the law
_____ mortified

_____ hurting myself and others
_____ liberated
_____ very strong
_____ a contortionist
Fantasies are _____ (more) _____ (less) important to most people than to me.

People I'd share safer sex fantasies with

_____

_____

_____

People I wouldn't share safer sex fantasies with

_____

_____

My sexual fantasies sometimes involve:

_____ being seduced
_____ getting fucked
_____ fucking
_____ watermelons
_____ animals
_____ sucking cock
_____ teasing
_____ eating pussy
_____ being raped
_____ feet
_____ raping
_____ group sex

_____ my priest, rabbi, gynecologist, policemen, and
_____ , and _____

_____ getting spanked

_____ spanking

_____ being in love

_____ fisting

_____ children

_____ men _____ women _____ both at the same
time

_____ King Kong and Fay Wray

_____ rimming

_____ being licked

_____ safe sex

_____ bondage

_____ watching others have sex

_____ cucumbers

_____ scat

_____ relatives

_____ massage

_____ Marilyn Chambers or Johnny Wad

_____ using a condom

_____ being the sex I'm not

_____ water sports

_____ tropical islands

_____ riding horses

_____

_____

_____

_____

My most common sexual fantasy goes like this:

_____

_____

_____

_____

_____

_____

_____

_____

_____

_____

_____

_____

_____

Here's the hottest safer sex fantasy I've ever had!

Write a SAFER SEX fantasy. You could make up an entirely new fantasy or you might rewrite the fantasy you created ABOVE. If your first attempt was a safe sex fantasy, you could opt to expand and elaborate the original creation.

If you use latex, nonoxynol-9, and/or other AIDS barrier techniques, consider lingering over this part of your fantasy. How do they get introduced into the sexual scene? What do these substances feel like, taste like, smell like? What does your partner think about them?

_____

_____

_____

_____

_____

_____

_____

_____

Final draft

After your first draft, look over your fantasy and ask yourself, "What would make this possible sexual encounter still safer *and* more exciting, hot, fun? What would make it riskier?" Then write the final draft.

_____

_____

_____

_____

_____

_____

_____

_____

_____

_____

_____

Total Body Masturbation

A basic component of good sex (both with ourselves and others) is good communication. In order to clearly communicate our sexual concerns, needs and desires, we must first know what they are. Masturbation is a great way for us to discover the language and responses of our own particular body. It is also an ideal way to show our partner(s) the kind of touching, stroking and timing we like and all the parts of our body that help to intensify our pleasure. Masturbation is also a safe and easy way for us to explore new ways of:

- Reaching sexual fulfillment
- Lengthening our orgasms
- Intensifying our orgasms
- Discovering the erotic potential of our entire body
- Discovering what turns us on and what turns us off
- Playing with multiple orgasm potential (yes, even for men!)

Masturbation time is also the time to become condom-conscious and proficient, and to get past any initial unfamiliarity, discomfort and resistance. It is a safe space:

- to learn what it takes to break a condom
- to discover the difference between them and which ones you like the best
- to find out how they can increase sensitivity and erotic pleasure

- to become very clear about what happens when you use an oil-based lubricant as opposed to a water-based one.

Remember, it's a lot safer to break a condom or make a mistake while playing outside the body than inside!

Give yourself permission to play with your body sexually and learn from it, even if you have never masturbated before. The following exercises are some ways you can use total body masturbation to help create a safer sex lifestyle.

Self Assessment—*Me and my masturbation, masturbation and me.*

Let's start with a masturbation assessment:

- How do you feel about masturbation?
- Where do you masturbate?
- When do you masturbate?
- Why do you masturbate?
- How do you masturbate?
- How frequently do you masturbate?

This is how I feel about masturbation—Check all that apply.

_____ it's a wonderful gift I can give myself

_____ it's a great way to have a quick orgasm or two, or more

_____ it's something only kids do

_____ it's healthy

_____ it will make me go blind

_____ only men masturbate

_____ it makes hair grow on my palms

_____ it's safe sex

_____ it's better than a partner

_____ it's more fun alone

_____ I feel guilty about masturbating

_____ People don't approve of me masturbating, such as:

    _____ my mom, _____ dad,

    _____ spouse, _____ lover,

    _____ friends, _____ minister,

    _____ Miss Manners, _____ the

hunk down the street,

    _____ my landlady, _____ my children, or

    _____ , _____ , _____

_____ it can increase my libido

_____ it can decrease my libido

_____ it's great for foreplay only

_____ it's something I'd like to get more out of

_____ must lead to orgasm

_____ is a way I can take responsibility for my own orgasms

_____ doesn't work for me

_____ is something I'd never admit to doing

_____ is something I like to watch other people do

_____ can't give me AIDS

_____ is a waste of time

_____ drains my energy

_____ is a great tension reliever

_____ is a sin

_____ is selfish
_____ is sexually liberating
_____ makes me feel secure, _____ sexy,
_____ ashamed, _____ embarrassed,
_____ happy, _____ angry,
_____ depressed, _____ neurotic,
_____ neutral

This is where I masturbate.

_____ in my bedroom, _____ with the lights out,
_____ door locked, _____ window shades drawn,
_____ covers over my head, _____ silently
_____ on the toilet _____ in the shower
_____ in the bathtub _____ at work,
_____ school, _____ library,
_____ movie-theater, _____ friend's house,
_____ in church _____ at Jack Off Parties
_____ in the swimming pool _____ doctor's office
_____ in front of the TV _____ where someone can catch me
_____ outdoors _____ in the warm sand,
_____ grassy meadow, _____ snow bank,
_____ mossy tree trunk, _____ at the water's edge
_____ on the train, _____ plane,
_____ bus, _____ horseback

This is when I masturbate.

_____ at night before falling asleep
_____ in the morning when I first wake up

_____ when I'm horny

_____ NEVER

_____ when I read or watch porn

_____ when no one's around

_____ when I have my period

_____ after partnered sex

_____ when I'm ovulating

_____ when I'm having an erotic dream in my sleep

_____

_____

_____

And here's WHY I masturbate!

_____ it feels so good

_____ it turns me on

_____ it's the only way I can have an orgasm

_____ it's the best way for me to have one

_____ I don't have a partner and can't afford to/won't
pay for sex

_____ it's a good release for my attraction to people
who are inaccessible or inappropriate

_____ I'm afraid of catching AIDS or other STDs

_____ my partner is unavailable

_____ it relieves tension, _____ boredom,
_____ anxiety, _____ stress,
_____ the jitters, _____ insomnia,
_____ blue balls

_____ it is good for my well-being

_____ it is part of my daily maintenance program

_____ I know my body better than anyone else

_____ it turns my lover on

_____ I have AIDS, _____ ARC,

       _____ have tested positive, _____ am in a high risk group and masturbation is the only thing I feel comfortable doing to protect my partner(s).

_____ I was told not to masturbate by

       _____ my parents, _____ doctor,

       _____ minister, _____ ex-partner,

       _____ teacher, _____ the pope,

       _____ and _____ .

_____ I start thinking about all this stuff and it makes me horny

How do I masturbate—let me count the ways.

_____ with my finger, _____ fingers,

_____ hand, _____ hands,

_____ feet,

_____ dry, _____ lubricated,

_____ my own lubrication _____ lube from a tube,

_____ with condoms, _____ dry,

_____ lubricated, _____ ribbed,

_____ smooth, _____ colored (which color(s),

_____ , _____

_____ latex, _____ naturals,

_____ with talcum powder inside,

_____ more than one at a time to create more sensation, friction and a harder hard-on

_____ using leather, _____ silk,

_____ latex, _____ feathers,

_____ clothes pins

_____ rubbing on the bed, _____ pillow,

_____ blanket, _____ rug

_____ with my vibrator(s), _____ externally,

_____ internally, _____ vaginally,

_____ anally, _____ on my genitals,

_____ breasts, _____ scrotum,

_____ thighs, and _____

_____ , _____

_____ with an acu-jack _____ dildo(s)

_____ water pick, _____ shower hose,

_____ faucet _____ liver,

_____ melon, _____ powder puff,

_____ the table leg _____ by squeezing my thighs together

_____ pinching my nipples _____ pulling my hair

_____ playing with my asshole _____ stimulating my prostate

_____ by using a hard stroking motion, _____ soft,
_____ fast,

_____ slow stroking motion

_____ on my partner's body

_____ between and/or on his/her thighs,

_____ breasts, _____ ass cheeks

_____ with my mouth _____ by fantasy alone

_____ while making a video of myself

_____ listening to Kate Smith sing

_____ smelling my partner's underpants

_____ licking his/her arm pits
_____ eating pizza

How often do I masturbate?

- To be perfectly honest, I masturbate

_____ never _____ 1 time,
_____ 2 times, _____ 3 times,
_____ 4 times, _____ a lot more times,
PER
_____ week, _____ month,
_____ day, _____ hour,
_____ year!

- And this is _____ too much, _____ too little, _____ just right for me.

Now that you know what you're doing, is there anything new you'd like to try? If so, here are some suggestions.

Creative Safer Sex Masturbation

Cheating AIDS by getting MORE out of our old-time favorite

Masturbate or pleasure your body in new ways—new position, a different hand, at a different time of night or day, with a new toy, with condoms, with new kinds of strokes, touching different parts of your genitals than you

177

usually do—however you like. Take lots of time for yourself. You need not have an orgasm or ejaculation. Try out using both hands, one on your genitals and the other somewhere else, at the same time. Close your eyes and try to get in touch with stroking both places simultaneously. As you do this, breathe slowly and evenly. Imagine the breath flowing along a path between the two places you are touching and stroking. See if this helps expand your sexual experience. Don't forget your anus. Relax. Explore. (Don't put anything in your vagina that has been in your anus without cleaning it first.) If you USUALLY don't want to masturbate your genitals, explore other parts of your body. As you pleasure yourself, explore safer sex fantasies. You might think about the fantasy you wrote, or something new. Don't strive for ideas, just let them very gently come and go during the exercise. If you are unable or don't want to have fantasies while masturbating, set aside time before or after this exercise for safe sex day dreams.

When you have finished the exercise, get into a comfortable position and reflect for about 10 minutes on the experience. How was it for you? What did you enjoy? What did you dislike? What would you like to do again?

Masturbation with Teasing, Smelling, and Tasting

Here are some ways to expand the enjoyment of masturbation. You may pick and choose as you like and are encouraged to add as many new details as you wish. Do this for approximately one hour.

This exercise will assist you in learning how your body feels at the different stages of arousal. Learn to build up sexual pleasure, then let it subside. Become aware of the feelings, relax a little, and then continue. This is known as *teasing*.

Masturbate until you feel your breathing increase, until you feel like going very fast, until you experience wanting to thrust your pelvis. Then stop and experience these feelings for awhile. Do not aim for an orgasm. Take a short break, one or two minutes.

Now begin again to stimulate yourself, using light stroking. Incorporate the Kegels you have learned. When there is sufficient lubrication in your vagina, or when you notice a secretion from the penis, take a few moments to smell and taste your own secretions. It's perfectly okay to like your own body juices *and* you will never get AIDS from your own body. If you are into same sex relations your own lubrication, smells and cum can be a wonderful enrichment to fantasy as well as a hot substitution for the sex juices of your partner(s). After you have teased yourself two or three times you may wish to rest, go on, or do something else.

Learning to Prolong Orgasm and Have Multiple Orgasms

While masturbating, watch how your body responds as you near climax. Do you hold your breath? Do you throw your head back? Do you tense and contract your pelvis and anal sphincter? If a male, do your testicles rise up close to your penis just before ejaculation? Do you hold your testicles up to cum faster? These are very common elements people experience in the preorgasmic stage of sex.

To intensify this plateau, experiment with changing your regular pattern:

- If you tend to hold your breath just before orgasm, try slow, deep breathing instead!
- If your neck is tensing and you want to throw it back, concentrate on relaxing your neck muscles and not throwing your head back.
- If you tend to lift your pelvis and/or contract your anus, try relaxing or even pushing down on the floor of your pelvis. Try pushing down with your anal sphincter as though you wished to defecate.
- If a male, experiment with relaxing your testicles when you notice they are rising and circle your scrotum above your testicles and gently pull them down. You might even want to hold them down for awhile. You can repeat this many times to prolong sexual pleasure.
- Remember you can also stop, change positions and techniques to prolong the process of orgasm.

Many people find that when they change their usual pattern of having an orgasm that the intensity and duration of orgasm increases dramatically.

Many people, especially men, assume that they are not multiply orgasmic. Often they have not tried continuing sexual activity after initial orgasm. There is even a myth that people should stop and be fulfilled by just one orgasm. Many women have been told they are incomplete if they aren't multi-orgasmic, when in fact they might be totally satisfied with one or none. Be your own judge. When using the techniques described above, people often find that with duration of orgasm comes the desire and ability to have more sexual activity. Men often find they maintain an erection and sexual intensity which enhances the possibility of having multiple orgasms.

Masturbation is a particularly good place to become experienced at these techniques. In addition, you might want to talk with your partner or friends. Teach them some of the ways you're learning to have a better time and ask how they make orgasms stronger or better.

This is how some of my friends make orgasms stronger and hotter:

_____

_____

Having Orgasms In Places Other than the Genitals

Many people rely entirely on their genitals for sexual gratification (this is especially true for men). Indeed, it

181

comes as a shock to many such people that it is often possible to have orgasms in other parts of the body which are sometimes as enjoyable, exciting and powerful as genital ones. This fact is well known to those who have lost their genital functioning for various reasons, and have had to look elsewhere on their bodies for orgasmic satisfaction. In fact, some adults who have lost all genital sensation due to spinal chord injuries report that the newly discovered and developed erotic parts of their bodies create orgasms more powerful and satisfying than any they can remember before their injury.

While learning to have orgasm(s) in nongenital parts of the body will be easier for some and impossible for a few, everyone can learn to increase and intensify the erotic potential and sexual response of other parts of the body. Having this option is important in creating a safer sex lifestyle. A side benefit of increasing our nongenital sexual potential is that in addition to having terrific sex without exchanging body fluids, we can have a wonderful time safely masturbating in social situations which otherwise would be boring, unpleasant or wasted time. Just be careful not to start moaning and groaning inappropriately!

Getting Started

To start exploring and developing nongenital erogeny, it is useful to remember that we invalidate what we are experiencing sexually in three different ways:

- By comparing our experience to what others are experiencing. "S/he seems to be enjoying this more than I am. I must be doing it wrong."
- By comparing our experience to past experiences. "I'm not getting aroused as quickly as when I

  _____ , _____ , _____

  therefore this is not okay."
- By comparing our experience to our expectation. "I thought I'd be having orgasms every time I squeezed my nipples hard. What am I doing wrong?"

Forget about what you used to think was true about you and your orgasm(s) and be willing to experience something extremely new. You may just surprise yourself.

Experiment any way you want to. Below are some guidelines that others have found very useful in developing new orgasmic potential.

Find a time when you can spend longer than you usually do for your "private time," maybe a couple of hours or the whole morning, afternoon or night. Find or buy some new things for your erotic enjoyment—satin sheets, candles, perfume, incense, feathers, oils, erotic porn, stirring music—something you haven't ever tried before. Surely there must be something! Set the stage for yourself. Take a slow bath or shower, really enjoying feeling your entire body as you bathe. Next do your sensory exercises or some yoga. Wake up all parts of your body.

Now invite yourself into your special environment.

Smell, touch, breathe, feel, breathe, look, listen, breathe. All the elements in your environment should be an erotic delight for you.

Find a comfortable spot, lay back, relax, breathe. Take your time!

- allow yourself to start fantasizing
- deepen your breath
- do your Kegels
- breathe
- begin stroking your body, caress your cheek
- explore your ears, squeeze your nipples, tug your hair
- do your Kegels
- breathe
- do more touching
- feel the skin between your toes, in your arm pits, under your chin, over your lips (take time)
- slowly move your finger tips over your body so lightly that you are playing with the point that they contact your skin and the point that they don't touch it
- breathe, enjoy
- find a nongenital part of your body that feels especially good
- now increase your stroking and pressure there
- now find another place and yet another
- intensify your Kegels, breathing, pressure and fantasies
- continue at your own pace playing, experimenting,

pleasuring your body; vary the speed and intensity of your breath, Kegels, fantasies, touching, stroking, caressing, petting, pinching, pulling, tugging, slapping, tapping.

Don't get caught up in searching for an orgasm. This is supposed to be pleasurable. If you do begin to have an orgasm, let it happen but don't stop pleasuring yourself. Remember, exploring and pleasure are the goal. You may find the orgasm continues beyond initial spasms, grows stronger, turns into multiple orgasms or fizzles quickly. If you *don't* have an orgasm during this exploring, increasing sensory awareness, and having fun with ourselves is the goal! Our *body* is the canvas, our *breath* is the paint, our *mind* the brush and we are the artists. ***Create!***

Experimenting with Condoms and Latex Gloves

- Buy as many different kinds of condoms as you can find and a few latex or neoprene examination gloves. The gloves can usually be found at the pharmacist's booth of drug stores and are sold singly or in pairs. They are also sold in boxes of 50 or 100 at surgical supply stores.
- Compare your latex treasures in terms of smell, taste, texture, elasticity, ease of opening, lubrication and durability.

- Play with them in a nonsexual context—put them on your feet, hands, genitals—put baby powder or talc inside and notice the difference that makes. Blow them up.
- Experiment with oil-based lubricants. Notice that they break down the latex, whereas water-based lubricants don't!
- During masturbation, blow a condom or latex glove up and tie a knot in the end. Condoms can be made to take the shape of not only penises but also female breasts! Smell, suck and lick your toy. Brush it over your nipples, breast, thighs, the lips of your vulva, your scrotum.
- For men, place a condom on your erect cock and try different kinds of water-based lube. Remember that initially you may experience a decrease in sensation or be constantly aware that having on a condom feels differently than not having on one.
- Let it be okay to have a different kind of feeling. Experiment with different kinds of condoms—how does each feel and which do you like best? Why? Try putting talc on the inside of a condom and lube on the outside. Try turning ribbed ones inside out (being careful to get all the air out when you put it on). Try wearing two condoms at the same time and notice what happens.
- Both men who have sex with men and women who have sex with men can get used to putting condoms on a partner by practicing with a dildo, zucchini or cucumber.

Let's Do Some Advanced Masturbation

Continue exploring creative masturbation. Be sure to include whole-body touching while masturbating—work out from the genitals, spreading the sexual energy throughout the whole body.

Incorporate breathing into your masturbation. It may be awkward at first, but give it a good try and see how it effects your sexual response, the strength and feel of your orgasm(s) and ejaculations. As you near orgasm, be sure to breathe deeply, do pelvic thrusting and Kegels. Concentrate on your pelvis. If your pelvis is lifted and contracted, see what purposefully relaxing it and then pushing down feels like—does it heighten your arousal, prolong your orgasmic plateau, help you feel sexual excitement deep within your vagina, make your clitoris more sensitive, your penis harder or have some other effect? If your pelvis is relaxed, what does it feel like to lift and contract your pelvic girdle, your ass hole, your pubococcygeus (Kegel) muscles.

Women, try putting a condom on your finger(s) and stimulating your genitals, or using a condom on a dildo or vibrator. Blow up a condom or rubber glove to the size you want to put in your vagina and tie a knot in the end. See how much softer and "flesh like" your new toy is. Tie knots in a condom and use them like Benwa balls. Snap and flap the latex gently on your genitals.

Men, try using condoms while masturbating, breaking some and trying out different brands. See how water-soluble lubricants affect the way rubbers feel and perform. Remember to change positions a lot, stroke the entire penis, including the part between the balls and the anal sphincter.

Keep breathing deeply and do something new with your asshole—gently stroke the outside part or leave it alone for a change, or carefully put something on or in it, maybe use a latex glove to play with it. Notice how much smoother the glove is than bare fingers and how it prevents pinching the intestinal walls with fingernails. You could tantalize the outside of your asshole with a piece of silk, velvet, latex or leather. It's up to you.

Sharing Masturbation with Others

Although most people masturbate, we have been taught to be secretive about masturbation. However, if we talk with others who are willing to share their experience, we often feel better about masturbation and learn many new ways to pleasure ourselves. SHARE the information you have learned about your masturbation and experimentation. Find out how other people feel about theirs. This can be in a sexual or nonsexual context with your spouse, lover, friend or support group.

Try out the following exercise:

Choose a partner with whom to share information about your mastubatory patterns. The questions below will help clarify your own views and attitudes as well as give you an opportunity to understand another point of view. Decide who will ask the question first and who will answer. When you have gone completely through the list, change roles.

- What is the earliest self-pleasuring you can remember?
- When did you first associate self-pleasuring with masturbation?
- How did you learn to masturbate? (self-discovery, friend, etc.)
- When did you have your first conversation about masturbation?
- How did you feel about masturbation as a teenager?
- How do you feel about masturbation now?
- What is your current pattern? How do you masturbate and how do you feel about it?

Safer Sex With Others

Communication Skills

By the time you finish this book, you will have a lot of information about yourself and safer sex. All that information will be of no use unless you can communicate it to your partner. Remember earlier in the chapter we said that sex was basically about communication? The following exercises are designed to help you develop safe sex communication skills.

Keep in mind that feelings of love and concern alone

do not insure we will have safe sex nor do they provide a blanket of protection against the possible consequences of unsafe sex. Knowledge and good communication create safety. They also create the foundation for strong, growing relationships.

Make Safer Sex Check Lists

It is a lot easier to make decisions at a safe, nonsexual time than in the heat of passion. Think about what might happen if you had sex with another person or people. Now create three lists: a YES list, a NO list, and a MAYBE list.

YES LIST. Write down all the things you feel comfortable doing with another person that are safe.

NO LIST. Now put down all the unsafe things you clearly do not intend to do.

MAYBE LIST. Here enumerate the things you're not sure about that depend on the partner and the situation.

Keep updating these lists and re-evaluating them.

Comparing Lists

Choose a partner to do this next exercise with who has made their own YES, NO, MAYBE list, your lover, spouse, someone you're dating or would like to date, a friend, or anyone who is adventurous and into improving their safe sex communication skills. A major purpose of the exercise is to strengthen your ability to hold to your resolve under all kinds of conditions.

- Pick something you feel strongly about from your YES list.
- Have your partner pick out something they feel strongly about from their NO list.
- Don't tell each other what you've picked.
- Stand face-to-face.
- For two or three minutes, convince your partner to do what you feel is okay just by saying yes while they try to convince you not to do what they don't want to do just by saying no.
- Shout, cajole, pout, look menacing, cold, irresistible, BUT you can only say one word: YES, and your partner can only say NO.
- Reverse roles. You pick something from your NO list and your partner picks something from their YES list and try to convince one another by your saying *only* NO and your partner only saying YES.
- Now repeat the whole exercise with you on your knees and your partner standing (both yes and no).
- Now do the exercise again only this time with you standing and your partner kneeling.
- Share with your partner what that was like for each of you and the feelings the exercise may have produced.
  ‡ This exercise becomes even more powerful in a support group with the whole room full of partners shouting "YES" and "NO" at the same time.
- ‡‡ It may be empowering to realize that "No." is a complete statement.

Share Your List

- Share your YES, NO, MAYBE lists with someone. Talk about why those particular things are in each list that they are.
- With someone you don't intend to be sexual with, practice negotiating what the two of you could do if you were going to be sexual. Are there parts of your list that are easier to negotiate than others?

Talking and Listening

Often there are times when we do not express our real feelings about AIDS or risk reduction to our partners because we don't know how our partners will react, or we are afraid of how they won't react. It is often especially difficult to convey negative feelings.

The purpose of this exercise is to provide each of you an open "safe" space in which to express your feelings about something, and to provide the assurance that you have been heard.

Ask your partner to read the rules of this communication exercise. Arrange with your partner to set aside a twenty-minute period in which to do this exercise.

Decide who will be the talker (A) first. The talker (A) talks for five minutes about something that he/she has feelings about, using statements beginning with "I" such as "I want," "I feel," "I do," "I am," as much as possible and avoiding statements like "you always," "you want," etc. The listener (B) may not interrupt except to ask for clarification, for example, "Could you be more specific?" When the talker (A) is finished, the listener (B) says "thank you" (for sharing that information). Then talker (B) begins to talk for five minutes. The listener (A) may not interrupt. If the second talker (B) wishes to make a comment about what (A) said during those five minutes, that's okay as long as the talker sticks to her/his own feelings on the subject. (A) says "thank you" when (B) is finished.

Many people find it helpful to wait at least twenty-four hours before responding with anything other than "thank you." After the first round, don't talk about that subject for a couple of hours or negotiate for another subject. Some of your negotiation with your partner can include deciding whether to take on a nonsexual or a sexual topic.

Role Plays

One of the best ways to prepare for real life situations is to practice and act out possible scenes and situations we face. In the following exercises, try out new situations, possibilities, and selves. Afterward, compare experiences with your partner(s). What worked and what didn't work? How could it have gone better? Do we want to practice again? How about changing roles?

Since we haven't spent much time on the AIDS antibody test, we will focus on this as an issue. Feel free to create your own role plays.

1. Two men are in a sexual relationship, one gay, one bisexual (also in a relationship with a woman). One tests negative and the other tests positive. They discuss how to tell their other partners.
2. A woman and a man are in a sexual relationship. The man used to share needles but won't take an antibody test.
3. Two women are in a sexual relationship, one bisexual and one lesbian dealing with issues of other partners who may be men.
4. You have just taken the test and haven't heard results yet.
5. You won't take the test for political and civil rights reasons, but a partner is trying to persuade you.
6. Two people, one tested negative, one positive, are still dealing with fear and the possibility of a false negative or false positive.

How To Say You Want To Play Safely

In our society, one of the hardest things to do for many people is to talk about sex. It seems that many of us believe that sex should be a spontaneous act where the communication just mystically happens. Unfortunately, it rarely seems to happen that way.

The first step in living a safer sex lifestyle is to make an agreement with yourself that you will only have sex if it is safer sex. Once that is clear, you only need to make sure that your partner is in agreement. If your partner is not willing to play safe, then you have to question whether this person is so hot that you are willing to risk death for a hot night at best. While that may be a bit overdramatic, it may be the best way of thinking about it.

So now that you have decided that you want to play safe, how do you get agreement from your partner? Listed below are a few lines that can be used in most situations to indicate that you want to play safe:

You do play safe don't you?

I think you are going to be my hottest safe sex partner ever.

What's your favorite brand of condom?

I only play safe.

I want you in that safe sex way.

I can't wait to rap my mouth around your condom clad rod.

I don't play unsafe.

How many condoms do you have?

Do you use the flavored dental dams?

I can hardly wait to lick your body thru my dental dam.

The only sex I do is safer sex.

Safer sex is where it is at for me.

I love it when you talk safer sex to me.

I love it when you do safer sex to me.

I love safer sex.

I used to do unsafe sex, but now I'm hotter.

I only say yes to safer sex.

The Complete Guide to Safer Sex

It's hotter with safer sex.
Unsafe sex turns me off.
Safer sex turns me on.
I'm hot for safer sex.
What really turns me on is safer sex.
Only if it's safe.
Do safe sex to me.
Yes, but only safer sex.
No, unless it's safe.
Do it to me! But do it safely.
My middle name is Safer Sex.
I want you, safely.
I'm steaming for some safer sex with you.
I'm so hot for safer sex with you.
I want to lick you, safely.
I want to ball your brains out, safely.
Take me, I'm yours, but do it safely.
I can hardly wait to get the condoms out.
I look at you and can only think about safer sex.
I won't do it unsafely.
I look at you with safer sex in my eyes.

The preceding are just a few ideas. Why don't you take a minute and write down some of your own.

_____
_____
_____
_____
_____

If They are Resistant

Unfortunately, some people do not want to play safely. It is difficult to say no to the person of your dreams just because they don't want to play safe. So here are some ways to counter their arguments:

I want sex to be spontaneous. You say fine as long as you can spontaneously put condoms and nonoxynol-9 lube on them. Then just do it. The lube and the condoms should be by the bed, the couch, in the car, at the office, anyplace you might have sex and plenty of the places where you wouldn't even think of it. Then, spontaneously, you can reach for your safe sex gear. You can put the condom on your partner, or put in your partner's diaphragm, or spread the nonoxynol-9 on your partner as the action proceeds.

I hate the taste of latex. You respond, "Not to worry, we get to try the ice cream in the fridge and the whipped cream, and if you're good maybe I'll throw in the cherry." Don't forget that some condoms and dental dams are flavored, and oral sex is just one part of the whole oral experience.

I don't do safer sex. The best response is, "Why?" Talking to your partner is the best way to clear up communication problems, and a line like that is a conversation opener, not closer. Take advantage and explore what the real problem is.

It is just so messy. This is something like the old Woody Allen line, "Sex is dirty, but only if you do it right." In fact, safer sex need not be messy at all, and if you're doing it right, what a great mess to make.

It does not feel as good. The idea is not to recreate the same exact feeling as unsafe sex, but to create and have fun with the new sensations. You can always ask how often the person has tried safer sex. You have to try it at least three times before you get any idea. The first time you are probably too nervous to really be clear about what it feels like. The second time is really the first time, and it is difficult to make judgments based on the first time. So by the third time, you can get some idea about what it is really like.

Can't we do it without condoms just once? NO!!!

It is so much bother. Not if you do it right. Let me show you how to get into it.

I really can't feel anything. The question here is, when was the last time they used a condom? Condoms are thinner than ever and conduct heat and tactile sensations remarkably well. You can increase the feeling by placing a couple of drops of lube in the condom as well as on the outside. Also, even if the sensation was significantly reduced, this is often helpful to men who have a tendency to ejaculate too soon. It could help prolong sex, which can be a fun thing to do. It is also important to know that orgasm, while you are inside your partner, is not essential to a satisfying sexual encounter. There is nothing wrong with coming by masturbation (with or without the condom) after you have disengaged from each other.

I'm too zonked to even think about it. Probably the Number One reason that people who want to have safe sex don't is the use of alcohol and other drugs. This book is not part of the anti-drug war. The fact is that many people use drugs (and alcohol is a drug) and they often make poor decisions while under the influence. Being too out of it to know that you can't drive is no excuse in a DUI (Driving Under the Influence). Being too out of it to do safer sex is just as dangerous as a DUI. If you can't act responsibly then maybe you are too out of it to act sexually at all. If safe sex becomes second nature to you, then maybe you will wind up doing it in your sleep, so to speak.

Using Lists to Help One Another Create Safer Sexual Options

PART A

1. Make a list of safer sex activities you would like to try but haven't, and make a list of unsafe activities you would like to really concentrate on making safer or avoiding. Have your partner or friend make lists too.
2. Write down three ways you would be willing to change unsafe activities and still have the sexual encounter remain erotic.
3. Then list three things your partner (or friend) could

change to lower risk and have the sexual encounter be erotic.

PART B

After you and your partner or friend have written your lists individually, read your lists aloud to each other. Discuss the new things you have learned about yourself and your partner. Each of you should decide on one thing you are going to change. The TALKING AND LISTENING exercises format presented earlier in this chapter will be helpful in doing this section of the exercise.

Dating Skills

Some people are expert at dating, but many are not, especially people who have been used to meeting their sexual needs by having anonymous encounters. Good dating differs from "just getting together" in that the special time is planned. Like a gourmet meal, if the preparation was done well, the event flows with the kind of ease that adds to enjoyment and frees the participants to be more spontaneous during the event itself. Below are some tips on how to put together dates that work.

- Parts of a date should be collapsible, expandable and expendable. If you are happy where you are you can expand the time in a particular activity; if not, you can shorten or skip that part.
- Make dates open ended. Don't make having sex or not having sex the high point of the evening. Create

several possible ways to end the encounter. Have several endings ready that will help you and your partner(s) to have a good time however the evening goes. And be open to experimenting. Let go of the script for the date if something more interesting comes up.

- Dating is a time to explore, play, experiment and become intimate with another person. Acknowledge these aspects of dates. You might want to tell your partner(s) how you feel—happy, anxious, confident, excited etc. If you're exploring new forms of relating, dating, having sex: tell them, let them know you hope they'll be part of this adventure.

- If you want to know a person better, be sure to plan dates so that much of the time is spent interacting, talking and/or entertaining each other. Dates in which the central focus is a movie, a concert, or a ballgame can be lots of fun, but are not successful in creating the deep intimacy that spending time alone and focusing on each other does.

A Dating Exercise

Spend time in a comfortable position thinking about how to put together a date you would really like to have. It could be a real date, a fantasy date, or an intimate evening with a friend. Be sure to incorporate lots of risk reduction and be sure to eroticize the techniques.

If you are partnered, consider spending a specific amount of time together doing something special, unusual and intimate. Settled partners often forget the importance of continuing to date one another. Dates add zest and playfulness to relationships and create a chance to explore new sexual and relationship options.

If you do not have any prospective dates, consider spending special time with a friend who is willing to explore this experience with you. Get to know one another better. If you tend to be a talker, see what it is like to carefully listen more. If you are usually quiet, try out communicating clearly about how you feel and what's going on in your life.

Safe Touch, Body Mapping, Erotic Massage

Just as sexual desire is a natural response of the body, so is our need to be touched, held, made to feel loved, valued and protected. The following exercises are designed to help convey the kind of touch that feels safe for each of you right now. Be aware that these feelings will keep changing and do not assume that what was true last week, last year or just a few moments ago is true now. In other words, stay present.

Give yourself permission to find a place and time that feels safe, sensual, unhurried and fun. You and your partner are going to be doing a series of massages over the next few days. Let each massage take approximately the same amount of time: 30 minutes, an hour, or longer. People usually have two common concerns when it comes to giving and receiving a massage: "What if I get aroused?" and "What if I don't get aroused?" These concerns can be assuaged by reaching an understanding before the massage begins. You may wish to negotiate a nonsexual massage, an open ended massage or a massage as part of a sexual encounter. Recognize that we never have to act on our feelings and that it's alright to become aroused. Just be clear, ahead of time, about what your mutual limits are for that particular massage. Also recognize that men get erections without being sexually aroused and are sometimes sexually aroused but do not get an erection. Let it be okay with you for your body or your partner's body to respond with pleasure.

- Review the work that you have been doing since the beginning of this chapter.
- Get in touch with how you are feeling right now. If there is any discomfort or anxiety, do some deep breathing. Remember, this is supposed to be fun.
- Choose who will receive the first massage. Let's say it's you.
- Decide the kind of massage you would like to have. It could be a foot, neck, scalp, back, hand or total body massage with your clothes on or off, with your partner's clothes on or off.

This *first massage* is entirely for your pleasure alone. However, your partner never has to do anything that feels uncomfortable or threatening. It will also help you in giving direction, stating exactly what you want, and help your partner in following directions, doing only what you say to do. After you have gotten into a comfortable position, tell your partner:

- what kind of oil, cream or talc, if any, you prefer
- where to start: toes, shoulders, face, etc.
- the kind of pressure you want: harder, firmer, softer, feathery, etc.
- the kind of stroking you want: long and slow, short and circular, tapping with the finger tips, slicing with the sides of the hands, brushing with the toes, etc.
- when to add more oil, cream or talc
- when to move to another area
- whether or not to use the peacock feathers, ping pong paddle, fur gloves, pumice, scalp massager, hair dryer, etc.
- finally, when to stop.

Now that the first massage is over, discuss with your partner, in a supportive and loving way, what that was like for you. Was it hard to give directions? Were you distracted by worrying what he/she was thinking, feeling, or experiencing? Did you feel as though you were being listened to? Is this someone that you feel you can trust? Did you feel safe? How did your partner feel about the experience?

You may want to wait a few hours, a few moments or a few days between each massage, whatever feels right and works best for you or your schedule, but you do not want to break the continuity of the massages by allowing too much time to pass between them.

The *second massage* is the same as the first except that you and your partner are going to reverse roles. It is your turn to give the massage and follow instructions. Remember, even though this is for his/her pleasure, you don't have to do anything that doesn't feel right to you. Again, afterwards review the experience.

For the *third massage* you are going to once again massage your partner. However, this time it is going to be for your satisfaction. Try experimenting with different kinds of strokes. Combine them. Vary your pressure. Use your finger tips, hands, arms, elbows, eyelashes, chest, your whole body. Cherish the individual you are playing with. Incorporate whatever toys you may have around and discover the ones that are the most fun for you to use. Don't use any lubrication on one part of the body. Next apply some talc and savor the contrast. Wash your hands, dry them and apply some warmed oil to another part of the body. Relish the difference. Be creative and appreciate the experience. When you are through, once more, share what happened for you.

For the *fourth and final massage* (that's right, you guessed it) you are going to reverse roles and repeat the third massage. Now all you have to do is lay back, relax and let go. Give yourself permission to be totally receptive and remember that you have the right to stop anytime you are uncomfortable.

After you and your partner have evaluated this massage, go back and look at all four massages. What did you learn about yourself and your partner? What kinds of touching do each of you like the best? Which massage was the easiest for you to do? Which was the most enjoyable, the hardest, the most relaxing? Which one would you like to repeat?

This next exercise is designed to see how much information you and your partner have learned about each other's sensual and erotic responses. On a large sheet of paper draw a treasure map of your partner's body. Circle the areas that are the most responsive. Indicate the path from one area to another. Make your map as detailed as possible. Note the spots to be avoided or gone lightly over. Let your lines reflect the correct kind of touching that your partner prefers. Then share the map. How accurate were you? How accurate was your partner? Let this be a learning experience.

Sexual Encounters

- Negotiate with a possible sexual partner about adding new dimensions to your safer sex life. What about looking for nongenital ways to give each other new sexual thrills? What about playing with condoms, latex gloves, dildoes, water-based lubricants, rubber dental dams, or vibrators?
- If you and your partner come up with some exciting decisions, consider creating a safe sex playshop. To do this, get together all the ingredients you will need and create a sensuous environment. Agree to play and experiment all you want. Agree to stop anytime either of you becomes uncomfortable, or just go on to something else. You don't have to like or dislike anything. You don't have to do everything with only one partner.

Group Sex

- If you like group sex, throw a *Jack Off Party* or a *Jack And Jill Off Party!* Introduce some of the toys you've been experimenting with and invite your guests to bring some too. Masturbation parties are a wonderful way to test out condoms safely.

- In fact, some people like to throw *Condom Testing Parties* as a separate event that includes any and all of the lowest risk sexual activities: masturbation, rubbing between the legs, on the body—you know, all the good stuff we've been covering so far!

After the party, talk with the other participants about how things went. What did they like the most? What was a turn off? What could be better next time?

S/M: Exploring intense sensation.

The more creative, imaginative, dynamic and sensitive a lover you are the easier the challenge of safer sex is going to be for you.

Many people have a lot of strong feelings about sadomasochism (S/M), both positive and negative. S/M, as it is used here, refers to either the consensual eroticizing of power or the exploration of intense tactile sensation. The purpose of this section is neither to convince you to change your ideas or feelings about S/M nor to encourage or advocate experimentation or exploration with this behavior. It is also not designed to justify, defend, negate or endorse S/M, but rather to look at risk reduction and heightened safer sex awareness and responsibility for those people whom are already engaging in the consensual eroticizing of power or interested in it.

Those of us who have been exploring S/M consciously with a partner and/or within the context of a community or support group may have some advantage in detailing constructively, creatively, effectively and erotically with the realities of safer sex. We are already used to handling issues of negotiating, setting limits and being concerned with issues of safety. We also know that we are only as safe as the toys and equipment we play with and our knowledge of how to use and take care of them.

The Care & Feeding of New Toys

Condoms, latex gloves, the correct water-soluble lube, rubber dams and hydrogen peroxide are just other toys to learn how to use properly. Sensitizing and erotizing ourselves and our partner(s) to these elements is the challenge at hand. We are also aware of the importance of total body arousal. Genital orgasms, if they are even part of the scene, are not necessarily the focus, goal or the end of the erotic experience.

Convincing our partner(s) to play safely and/or use a condom can heighten and intensify our play. *"If you're a top, demand safer sex. If you're a bottom beg for it,"* has been the loving and playful advice of the Sexologist's Sexual Health Project and the San Francisco AIDS Foundation to the men and women in the S/M communities. Keeping the action hot is where it is at. Decide ahead of time how you are going to deal with the possibly unsafe tendencies of your friend(s) so you don't have to make those decisions in the heat of passion.

Remember, nothing will spoil a scene faster than a long, boring lecture on the mechanics of safer sex or the medical aspects of AIDS. That doesn't mean that we don't want to raise our partner's consciousness. Just keep instructions brief, direct, hot, playful, firm, hot, clear, to the point, hot, hot and hotter still. Have your bottom crawl to you, begging to put a condom on your big hard dick and don't let them use their hands. Make them use just their lips. Let your top know you can still give her head but use a rubber dam over her clit or a condom on your tongue. Learn how to do it so that no one can resist this sexy safe sex approach.

Latex Sensations
Give yourself permission to embrace latex as a new medium to be explored. If you go looking in fabric stores or mill outlets you can sometimes find large sheets of latex from bolt remnants. Because it easily sticks to itself there are a lot of creative clothes you can make out of it or you can wrap it around your partner, mummy-fashion.

The advantage of completely encasing someone in latex (plastic wrap will also work) is that now your playmate is protected and you are free to rub whatever body juices you want all over them and watch them squirm. In a short while you may notice that the contents of your "human baggie" will begin to get very warm and

209

sweat. A spanking in this condition creates an interesting sensation. Or, instead, you can decide which part of the package looks the most appealing and rip, shred, bite, tear or slowly peel that section of latex open and do whatever it is you do to heighten the tactile awareness in that one area.

Another latex baggie idea, if you think your bottom would appreciate the sensation, would be to slip an ice cube(s) into the bag and see how long it takes to melt. It might also be interesting to see if you can make the ice cube(s) move from one end of the bag to another just by using your: toes, lips, tits, dick, ass, stomach, nose, vaginal lips or whip, paddle, belt or chains. What happens to the content of the bag when they get excited and their sexual juices start to flow? Also any of the commercial plastic wraps make exciting rip-away bondage.

One of the joys of latex gloves is that prostatic massages and sticking your fingers into warm, wet, juicy orifices are once again a safe option, provided you are using a water-soluble lubricant and your nails are short and in good condition. Keep in mind that you want to change fingers and/or gloves if you go from one opening to another. That shouldn't present a problem since latex gloves can be bought reasonably in boxes of one hundred. Talc on the inside of the glove gives a unique feeling to your hand, especially if you're spanking someone's ass. In addition to wearing them, gloves can be used to slap and snap: over thighs, tits, asses, arms, dicks, balls, or anywhere else you can think of. The sooner we learn to appreciate the options available, the sooner we can recreate the lifestyle most appropriate to who we are. Many people report that having to come up with new ways of enjoying "old favorites" has made their sex life more exciting than it ever was before. It's all up to us.

Ass Play

Anal fisting, fist fucking, hand balling or internal massage refers to the insertion of the hand or forearm into the rectum. For many people into fisting this is the most erotic, euphoric, transcendental, loving and intimate form of sexual expression. It is also, however, one of the most potentially dangerous, especially if either or both parties have been drinking or using drugs or poppers. What makes fisting so extremely risky in relationship to AIDS is that the blood vessels in the rectum are very close to the surface and that the upper colon is lined with extraordinarily delicate tissue. Even in the most careful and relaxed situation, trauma can easily occur and go unnoticed.

In addition to that is the fact that the best kind of lubrication for fisting is a heavy oil-based one, like Crisco, which is the worst type in relation to safer sex. The problem is twofold. First, oil-based lube, as stated before, breaks down the latex in condoms and rubber gloves. Second, it provides the best medium for bacteria and viruses to be cultured. The other difficulty is that most water-soluble lubricants dry out faster than is

211

needed for the prolonged amount of time it takes to adequately fist someone.

If fisting is a part of your lifestyle that is important for you to continue, do not use drugs, alcohol, poppers or oil-based lubes. Use a very tender and gradual insertion of the hand and avoid excessive friction. Consistently wear a latex glove. Opera-length ones can be found in beauty supply stores. Horse condoms, which are used to collect the semen for artificial insemination when breeding race horses, can be gotten at a veterinary supply house. Never have anal intercourse before or after fisting unless a condom is used. Keep experimenting with different water-based lubes until you find the one that best works for you. While you are adjusting to using a latex glove during fisting, it is important to focus on new feelings and sensations. Do not be discouraged.

Vaginal Fisting

Vaginal fisting, the gradual introduction of the hand into the vagina or actually touching or holding the cervix in your hand and feeling the ballooning capacity of the vagina can be highly erotic for both the giver and the receiver. It presents less problems than anal fisting for several reasons. First, the blood vessels in the vagina are not as close to the surface as in the anus and the tissues are not as delicate as that of the upper colon. While women vary in the amount of vaginal secretions they have, the use of a heavy, thick lube is not as desirable. However, just as with anal fisting, it is important to always wear a latex glove, make sure that there is no danger of piercing the glove with a rough or sharp fingernail or hangnail, and never go from the anus to the vagina without changing gloves. A loving, careful and tender approach is what is needed during any kind of fisting.

Water Sports

Water sports, or golden showers refers to urinating on or in someone. Because there are blood cells which can transmit the virus in urine, pissing in is out. However pissing on is in as long as there are no cuts or abrasions on the skin. Watch out for athlete's foot. If that's a problem, put a condom or rubber glove on your foot (yes, they will stretch that much) and pee away. Some people have found that securing a condom to the base of the cock via a cock ring or leather thong allows them to pee into the condom while someone is watching at close range or to safely play with the contents.

Biting and Nibbling

Biting, nibbling, chewing and *scratching* are all sensuous and erotic behaviors that numerous people find stimulating and engage in, yet seldom think of as having anything to do with S/M. It is, nonetheless, behavior that is considered part of an S/M continuum. Frequently the same people who find black leather, whips and chains so offensive, think nothing of the unexpected bruises, scratches or "love hickies" on their bodies the morning after a particularly passionate sexual encounter.

Nibbling on ear lobes, necks or thighs; biting various body parts; chewing on elbows, ass cheeks, scrotum skin or toes; or gently scratching backs, legs, asses or arms are basically safe sex activities that present little or no risk of AIDS transmission. Still, you do want to watch out for scrapes or cuts that can create a condition for receiving unwanted body fluids. Make sure that in your excitement and abandonment you do not draw blood. If this does occur, especially on the genitals, immediately apply an antiseptic ointment or diluted hydrogen peroxide. The point is, you don't need to give up being passionate or hedonistic. Just be responsible for your actions.

Piercing

Piercing the ears has been acceptable for women for centuries and the norm among any Elizabethan males who could afford jewelry. Today it is increasingly popular with young gay, bi and straight men. Among the punk chic, multiple ear piercing is the fashion for both sexes. Prince Albert, Queen Victoria's husband, is claimed to have had his cock pierced through the urethra and a ring placed through it. Today, that particular style of piercing is actually called a Prince Albert. Those who engage in piercing as an erotic form of sexual expression claim that there is greater sensitivity to the nipple, labia, cock or what ever other area is pierced. Placing a gold or surgical steel ring or bar through the piercing adds to the sensation and increases visual eroticism for many. Sometimes it is also an act of submission in a mutual and consensual exchange of power.

On the other hand, piercing presents some concerns. In piercing, the skin is punctured and depending on how long a person's body takes to heal after a piercing, it is possible for any of these fluids to enter the body and transmit the virus if you are not careful. How ever long it takes for that part of the body to heal, leave it alone or make sure it is securely covered with latex.

The more serious problem is similar to that of sharing needles in intravenous drug use. If you are into piercing and want to continue without putting yourself or those you play with at risk, make sure that you always use sterilized equipment and never share it. The supplies involved are readily available and inexpensive, so everyone can have their own set. Frequently, in large cities, leather stores or tattoo parlors will perform the piercing safely for you. Check within the community and get the names of professional piercers who are AIDS aware (they will always use single-use needles, wear gloves, and keep their equipment sterilized). Probably the safest way to have it done, if not the most erotic, is to ask your physician to do it.

Phone sex

This is an excellent example of how some people have adapted to the current health crisis. It views sex as part of the solution rather than seeing it as "the problem." It also points .out what sexologists have been saying for years:

sex is more about what is happening between our ears than what is going on between our legs. Keep in mind that this refers to consensual behavior and is not to be confused with illegal, nonconsensual, harassing and obscene phone masturbation calls. Consensually listening to someone's hot, steamy, sexy voice on the other end of the telephone while you are getting off is not a new phenomenon. People have been doing this for years. However, it has never been as wide spread or as popular as it is today, nor have there been the wide range of commercial services that are currently available.

The following are just a few suggestions that have come from some of the participants in the Eroticizing Safer Sex workshops presented by the Sexologist's Sexual Health Project over the past ten years:

- Read your favorite erotic literature to your partner over the phone, in a deep sexy voice and practice your Kegels.
- Call your lover at a time they can't respond adequately (like when they are at work) and tell them, in as much graphic detail as possible, the parts of their body that drive you wild with desire, and why. Remind them to practice their Kegels.
- Late at night, plan an uninhibited weekend together over the phone. Be specific.
- Give someone instructions on how to masturbate just by talking to them over the phone.
- Pretend to be a new fantasy lover and describe yourself and what you would like to do to them if they

would only be willing to meet you right now in some dark secluded place!

- While you are talking to your partner on the phone, each of you begin to stroke yourself and imagine that your hand is theirs. Practice your Kegels.
- During a long, slow sensuous bath, call your paramour and whisper sweet nothings into his/her ear. Practice your Kegels.
- Order your lover to call you at a specific time and tell her/him how you want her/him dressed or undressed.
- Leave a sexually explicit message on their answering machine when you are sure they're the only one who will receive it.
- Give a slow verbal massage over the phone, and practice your Kegels.
- Together, call one of the sexually explicit phone services that are in abundance right now, and get ideas on how to spice up your own phone fantasy play.
- Call your lover and describe your favorite safer sex experiences or fantasies.
- If you are into group sex, consider making conference calls.

The possibilities are only as limited as your imagination. Give yourself permission to be imaginative and experimental. Get consent from anyone you would like to call and negotiate the parameter of your calls. Is it alright to phone in the middle of the night? Can I call you at work? Are there any fantasies that would be upsetting to you? What fantasies turn you on the most?

Be creative and have fun.

Seeking Professional Help

We all learn in a variety of different ways. Some learning modalities will make it easier for us to make the changes in our lives that we need to make and others will make it more difficult. Hopefully, reading this book and practicing the techniques suggested here will be of major benefit to most people. However, if you find that this is not true for you or your lifestyle in a way that works comfortably and joyously for you or you would like to make those changes faster, you might want to seek further help.

Find the nearest college or university to you that has a human sexuality program. Call them and get the names of several clinical sexologists or sex-positive therapists in your area. Interview each one to make sure that you feel comfortable with them and that they have worked through their own issues about AIDS and safer sex. Watch out for the counselor whose denial system is such that they minimize the problem, rationalizing that you are at greater risk just crossing the street than contacting the virus and leaving you feeling that all you need to do to be safe is to avoid sexual contact with gay or bisexual men or prostitutes. On the other extreme are the helping professionals who are so frightened that they suggest you stop being sexual or give up large and important aspects of your sexual behavior or lifestyle, like anal intercourse, swinging, french kissing, relating to men on a sexual basis, S/M, open relationships, etc.

After reading this book you probably have as much or more information about AIDS, AIDS transmission and safe sex as most doctors and counselors in the field. Information alone is not what you are seeking. What you want is a professional who can nonjudgmentally assist you through a Sexual Attitude Restructuring process (S.A.R.) and helps you in developing a sex-positive environment so that you can make the changes and develop a lifestyle most appropriate to who you are.

Once you have chosen someone, be specific about the concerns that are not working for you. There is little use in spending a great deal of time on the pros and cons of condom usage when what you are really worried about is how, when and where to even broach the subject of safe sex to anyone. Likewise, sexual communication skills are premature if you feel that sex equals death or that sperm is toxic. With your therapist, set realistic goals, objectives and a timeframe to work from.

If you do not have a partner or are afraid to experiment with someone who may have no more ability to handle safer sex interactions than you, your sex counselor may suggest the use of a sex surrogate. Surrogates are highly-trained members of a sex therapy program, and they can be extremely effective in helping you to:

- develop safer sex communication skills
- become comfortable with condom usage
- learn to eroticize other parts of your body
- incorporate safer sex techniques into the things you already like to do sexually
- empower the options available to you
- feel sexual again
- be playful sexually
- get past your resistance to safe sex on a physical level.

At the same time, your therapist will be assisting you to:

- look at the emotional feelings that emerge for you between each session
- identify sex-negative messages and
- replace them with positive and reaffirming ones
- validate your right to be sexual, even in the Age of AIDS
- notice resistance on an emotional level and
- discover ways of working through your resistance
- clarify sexual preferences
- transfer what you have learned from the surrogate to your partner(s) or potentional partner(s).

There are many people within the medical profession who have a lot of strong judgmental feelings about unorthodox sexual practices. It is your responsibility to carefully choose a healthcare provider that you feel you can trust and to be able to sort out potentially lifesaving advice from sex-negative biases towards your lifestyle. Get the names of sex-positive doctors from friends within your community. You'll be glad you did.

FOOTNOTES

Chapter 2

1. For an excellent review see Curran, J.W., W.M. Morgan, A.M. Hardy, H.W. Jaffe, W.W. Darrow, W.R. Dowdle. "The Epidemiology of AIDS: Current Status and Future Prospects." Science 1985 September 27; Vol. 229. and Castro, K.G., A.M. Hardy, J.W. Curran. "AIDS and Other Medical Problems in the Male Homosexual: The Acquired Immunodeficiency Syndrome: Epidemiology and Risk Factors for Transmission." The Medical Clinics of North America 1968 May; 70(3), pp. 635–649.

Chapter 3

1. Centers For Disease Control: "Acquired Immunodeficiency Syndrome (AIDS) Update—United States." Morbidity and Mortality Weekly Report (MMWR), 1983 June 24; 32:309–11. Centers For Disease Control: "Acquired Immunodeficiency Syndrome (AIDS): Precautions for Health Care Workers and Allied Professionals." MMWR, 1983, Sept. 2; 32:450–452.

2. Friedland G.H., B.R. Saltzman, M.F. Rogers, P.A. Kahl, M.M. Mayers and R.S. Klein. "Lack of Transmission of HTLV-III/LAV Infection to Household Contacts of Patients with AIDS or AIDS Related Complex with Oral Candidiasis." The New England Journal of Medicine, 1986 Feb. 6; Vol. 314 No. 6, pp. 344–349.

also,

Gerald Friedland, Patricia Kahl, Brian Saltzman et al "Additional evidence for lack of transmission of HIV infection by close interpersonal (casual) contact" in AIDS 1990(4)7:639–644.

3. Acquired Immunodeficiency Syndrome (AIDS) in Western Palm Beach County, Florida. MMWR, 1986 Oct. 3; 35(39) pp. 609–612.

4. Castro, K., S. Lieb, C. Calisher, C. Schable, E. Buff, J. Witte, et al. Centers for Disease Control in Atlanta and Fort Collins, USA; and Florida Department of Health & Rehabilitative Services: "Seroepidemicologic Studies of HTLVIII/LAV Infection in Belle Glade, Florida." International Conference on AIDS, Paris 1986, Poster 685.

5. Centers for Disease Control: "Acquired Immune Deficiency Syndrome (AIDS): Precautions for Clinical and Laboratory Staffs." MMRW, 1982 Nov. 5; 31:577–80. Centers for Disease Control: "Acquired Immune Deficiency Syndrome (AIDS): Precautions for Health Care Workers and Allied Professionals. MMWR, 1983 Sept. 2; 32:450–452.

6. Centers for Disease Control: "Update: Prospective Evaluation of Health-Care Workers via the Parenteral or Mucosus-Membrane Route to Blood or Body Fluids from Patients with Acquired Immunodeficiency Syndrome—United States." MMWR, 1985 Feb. 22; 43:101—103.

7. Wofsy, C.B., J.B. Cohen, L.B. Hauer, N.S. Padian, B.A. Michaelis, L.A. Evans, J.A. Levy "Isolation of AIDS-Associated Retrovirus from Genital Secretions of Women With Antibodies to the Virus." The Lancet, 1986 Mar. 8; Vol. I. (8480) pp. 527–529.

8. "Genital Mucosal Transmission of Simian Immunodeficiency Virus: Animal Model of Heterosexual Transmission of Human Immunodeficiency Virus." C.J. Miller et al, Journal of Virology Oct. 1989(63)10:4277–4284.
Also see,
"Dendritic Cells Tapped as Ultimate HIV Reservoir" Anon. Clinical Immunology Spectrum, September 1991:3–4.

9. Salahuddin, S.Z., J.E. Groopman, P.D. Markham, M.G. Sarngadharan, R.R. Redfield, M.F. McLane, M. Essex, A. Sliski, R.C. Gallo. "HTLV-III In Symptom Free Seronegative Persons. The Lancet, 1984; 2:1418.

10. Groopman, J.E., S.Z. Salahuddin, M.G. Sarngadharan, et al. "HTLV-III in Saliva of People with AIDS Related

Complex and Healthy Homosexual Men at Risk for AIDS." Science 1984; 226:447–449.

11. Schecter, M.T., J.B. Boyko, E. Jeffries, B. Willoughby, R. Nitz and P. Constance. "The Vancouver Lymphadenopathy AIDS Study: 1. Persistent generalized lymphadenopathy." Canadian Medical Association Journal, 1985 June 1; Vol. 132, p. 1275.

12. Ho, D.D., R.E. Byington, R.T. Schooley, T. Flynn, T.R. Rota, M.S. Hirsch. "Infrequency of Isolation of HTLV-III Virus from Saliva in AIDS." New England Journal of Medicine 1985; 313:1606.

13. M.T. Schechter, W.J. Boyko et al. "Can HTLV-III Be Transmitted Orally?" The Lancet, 1986 February 15; p. 379.

14. Archibald, D.W., L. Zon, J.E. Groopman, M.F. McLane and M. Essex. "Antibodies to Human T-Lymphotropic Virus Type III (HTLV-III) in Saliva of Acquired Immunodeficiency Syndrome (AIDS) Patients and in Persons at Risk for AIDS." Blood, 1986 March; Vol. 67, No. 3: p. 831.

15. Chmiel, J., R. Detels, M. Van Raden, R. Brookmeyer, L. Kingsley, R. Kaslow and The Multi-Center AIDS Collaborative Study (UCLA, Los Angeles; NWU, Chicago; JHU, Baltimore: UP, Pittsburgh; NIAID, Bethesda). "Prevention of LAV/HTLVIII Through Modification of Sexual Practices." International Conference on AIDS, Paris 1986.

16. Tsoukas, C., T. Hadjis, L. Theberge, P. Gold, M. O'Shaughnessy, P. Feorino. "Risk of Transmission of HTLVI-II/LAV from Human Bites." International Conference on AIDS, Paris 1986, Poster 211.

17. Zon, L., D.W. Archibald, M.F. McLane, M. Essex, M.J. Hepner, J. Groopman. "IGA Deficiency and Salivary Transmission of Human Immunodeficiency." The Lancet, 1986 Nov.1; Vol. II. (8514) pp. 1039–1040.

18. Voeller, Bruce. "AIDS Transmission and Saliva." The Lancet, 1986 May 10; Vol. I. (8489) pp. 1099–1100.

19. Barr, C. E., J.P. Torosian. "Oral Manifestations in

Patients with AIDS or AIDS-Related Complex." The Lancet, 1986 Aug. 2; Vol. II. (8501) p. 288.

20. Vogt. M. W., D.J. Witt, D.E. Craven, R. Byington, D.F. Crawford, R.T. Schooley, M.S. Hirsch. "Isolation of HTLV-III/LAV from Cervical Secretions of Women at Risk for AIDS." The Lancet, 1986 Mar. 8; Vol. I. (8480) pp. 525–527.

Wofsy, C.B., J.B. Cohen, L.B. Hauer, N.S. Padian, B.A. Michaelis, L.A. Evans, J.A. Levy. "Isolation of AIDS-Associated Retrovirus from Genital Secretions of Women With Antibodies of the Virus." The Lancet, 1986 Mar. 8; Vol. I. (8480) pp. 527–529.

Vogt, M., D.J. Witt, D.E. Craven, R. Byington, R.T. Schooley, M.S. Hirsch. "Isolation of LAV/HTLV-III From Female Genital Secretion." International Conference on AIDS, Paris 1986, Communication 136:S30e.

21. Wofsy, C.B., J.B. Cohen, L.B. Hauer, N.S. Padian, B.A. Michaelis, L.A. Evans, J.A. Levy. "Isolation of AIDS-Associated Retrovirus from Genital Secretions of Women With Antibodies to the Virus." The Lancet, 1986 Mar. 8; Vol. I. (8480) pp. 527–529.

22. Centers for Disease Control: "Immunodeficiency among Female Sexual Partners of Males with Acquired Immunodeficiency Syndrome (AIDS)—New York. MMWR, 1983; 31:697–698.

Harris, C., C. B. Small, R. S. Klein, et al. "Immunodeficiency in Female Sexual Partners of Men With the Acquired Immunodeficiency Syndrome." New England Journal of Medicine, 1983; 308:1181–1184.

23. Pape, J. W., B. Liautaud, F. Thomas, et al. "Characteristics of the Acquired Immunodeficiency Syndrome (AIDS) in Haiti." New England Journal of Medicine, 1983; 303:945–950.

Pape, J., B. Liautaud, F. Thomas, et al. "The Acquired Immunodeficiency Syndrome (AIDS) in Haiti." Annals of Internal Medicine, 1985; 103:674–678.

Piot, P., H. Taelman, K.B. Minlangu, et al. "Acquired

Immunodeficiency Syndrome in a Heterosexual Population in Zaire." The Lancet, 1984; 2:65–69. Vande Perre P., P. Le Page, P. Kestelyn, et al. "Acquired Immunodeficiency Syndrome in Rwanda." Lancet, 1984; 2:65–69.

24. Kreiss, J.K., D. Koech, F.A. Plummer, K. King, M. Lightfoote, P. Piot, A. R. Ronald, J. O. Ndinya-Achola; D'Costa et al. "AIDS Virus Infection in Nairobi Prostitutes: Spread of the Epidemic to East Africa." New England Journal of Medicine, 1986 February 13; 314(7)pp. 414–418.

Bigger, R.J. "The AIDS Problem in Africa." The Lancet, 1986 Jan. 11; Vol. I (8472) pp. 79–82.

Mascart-Lemone F., M. DeBruyere, P. Vandeperre, J. Dasnoy, L. Marcelis et al. "Acquired Immunodeficiency Syndrome in African Patients." The New England Journal of Medicine. 1984 February 23; 310 (8) pp. 492–497.

25. Franzen C., M. Jeriborn, G. Biberfeld: "Four Generations of Heterosexual Transmission of LAV/HTLVIII in a Small Swedish Town." International Conference on AIDS, Paris 1986, Poster 199.

26. Wofsy, C.B., J.B. Cohen, L.B. Hauer, N.S. Padian, B.A. Michaelis, L.A. Evans, J.A. Levy. "Isolation of AIDS-Associated Retrovirus from Genital Secretions of Women With Antibodies to the Virus." The Lancet 1986 Mar. 8; Vol. I. (8480) pp. 527–529.

Kreiss, J. K., D. Koech, F. A. Plummer, K. King; M. Lightfoote, P. Piot, A. R. Ronald, J. O. Ndinya-Achola, D'Costa et al. "AIDS Virus Infection in Nairobi Prostitutes: Spread of the Epidemic to East Africa." New England Journal of Medicine, 1986 February 13; 314 (7) pp. 414–418.

27. Jaffe, H. W., K. Choi, P.A. Thomas, et al. "National Case-control Study of Kaposi's Sarcoma and Pneumocystis Carinii Pneumonia in Homosexual Men: Part 1, Epidemiologic Results." Annals of Internal Medicine, 1983; 99:145–151. 1983.

Marmor, M., A.E. Friedman-Kien, S. Zolla-Pazner, et al. "Kaposi's Sarcoma in Homosexual Men: A Seroepidemiologic

Case-control Study." Annals of Internal Medicine, 1984; 100:809–815.

Goedert, J., M.G. Sarngadharan, R.J. Biggar et al. "Determinants of Retrovirus (HTLV-III) Antibody and Immunodeficiency Conditions in Homosexual Men." The Lancet, 1984; 2:711–716.

APPENDIX

Heterosexual AIDS transmission did not begin to be studied in depth until the late 1980's due to the low number of cases in the United States and other social, political factors. The best work to date is *Heterosexual Transmission of AIDS* Eds. N.L. Alexander, H.L. Gabelnick and J.M. Spieler Wiley-Liss: NY 1990. Below is a synopsis of earlier important research findings.

1. In 1979, a Swedish sailor came down with acute symptoms of HIV infection about one month after sex with a female prostitute in Haiti. He returned to Sweden remaining symptom free but contagious. Three of his six female hometown sexual partners between 1979 and 1986 became infected with HIV. One of the women had sex with a married man between 1982 and 1985. The man became infected but his wife remained seronegative. The spouse of the seaman had symptoms of HIV infection in 1983, about one month after their first intercourse and was found to be antibody positive in 1985. Their son, born in 1985 is antibody positive. The researchers conclude:

Our investigation gives strong evidence for female-male and male-female transmission of LAV/HTLVIII in 4 generations, affecting at least 3 women in child-bearing age and 2 male partners, none of them belonging to established risk-groups.

Franzen, C., M. Jeriborn, G. Biberfeld. "Four Generations of Heterosexual Transmission of LAV/HTLVIII in a Small Swedish Town." International Conference on AIDS, Paris 1986, Poster 199.

2. Researchers at Walter Reed Army Institute studied 22 steady heterosexual partners of men and women with HIV infection. The couples had been in a sexual relationship for at least 2 years. Spouses of the infected patients all had no defined risk factor other than sexual contact with their partner. Eight

partners of the infected patients (2 men and 6 women) also became infected. Reporting on the sexual activities of the 22 couples, the researchers state:

> All 22 couples routinely engaged in vaginal-penile intercourse. Oral-genital sex was practiced to varying degrees by all the couples. Two uninfected contact wives reported occasional anal intercourse. More importantly, anal intercourse was denied by all the infected females. These data show frequent bi-directional heterosexual transmission of HTLVIII/LAV among couples who engage in recurrent vaginal-penile intercourse.

Redfield, R., D.C. Wright, R. Markham, S.Z. Salahyddin, R. Gallo, and D. Burke. "Frequent Bidirectional Heterosexual Transmission of HTLVIII/LAV Between Spouses." International Conference on AIDS, Paris 1986, Poster 207.

3. In another study consisting of 57 heterosexual partners of 52 patients with AIDS, researchers found that 36 partners (63%) have remained healthy while 21 (37%) have become infected with HIV (17 of 48 females and 4 of 9 males). One heterosexual partner developed AIDS, 7 came down with ARC and 8 have clinical abnormalities. However, the researchers were unable to ascertain the sexual activities which caused transmission:

> There were no significant associations between serologic status or clinical illness and duration of relationship, number of episodes of sexual contact, anal intercourse, sex with menses, other sexual practices, use of condom or diaphram, or serologic markers for CMV or Hepatitis B.

Saltzman, B., C.A. Harris, R.S. Klein, G.H. Friedland, P.A. Kahl, N.H. Steigbigel, et al. "HTLVIII/LAV Infection and Immunodeficiency in Heterosexual Partners (HP) of AIDS Patients." International Conference on AIDS, Paris 1986, Poster 210.

4. In another study of heterosexual partners of AIDS patients and household transmission, researchers found no household transmission among 109 children and 29 adult relatives of 45 AIDS patients; but found that 26 (58%) of the 45 spouses developed HIV antibodies—11 of 17 male partners and 15 of 28 female partners. Ten developed clinical manifestations of infection. Infection with gonorrhea and a positive test for syphilis correlated with HIV antibodies, while "Oral sex and lack of barrier contraceptives correlated with seroconversion."

Fischl, M.A., G.M. Dickinson, G.B. Scott, N. Klimas, M.S. Fletcher, W. Parks. "Heterosexual and Household Transmission of the Human T-lymphotrophic Virus Type III." 1986 International Conference on AIDS, Paris 1986, Communication 175.

GLOSSARY

Oh perish the use of the four-letter words
Whose meanings are never obscure!
The Anglos and Saxons, those bawdy old birds
Were vulgar, obscene, and impure.

But cherish the use of the weaseling phrase
That never quite says what you mean!
You'd better be known for your hypocrite ways
Than as vulgar, impure, and obscene.

The authors decided that the glossary of the Guide should be fun to read by itself, rather than just a dull list of words. It also should have an educative function, to explain and define concepts that may be foreign to us. To this end, we will give the colloquial equivalent(s) of the scientific (polite) terms and the scientific equivalent(s) of the colloquial (dirty) terms, wherever possible.

We have learned not to use "dirty" words in polite society. The polite terms can be either scientific or euphemisms, both of which can obscure the meaning. For example, the following except from a "trashy" novel, "I fucked her asshole doggie-style while squeezing her tits," loses something in its translation to "I engaged in rear entry anal coitus while applying pressure to her breasts." There is also power in the ability to use, hear, and understand colloquial terms.

As a last note, no glossary can be complete in so few pages.

GLOSSARY

Abstinence—Not taking part in sexual acts. Some people include masturbation in this definition, others do not. Some people use celibacy to denote this concept, but that actually means: to not marry (i.e. vow of celibacy). Asceticism is also used, but is more of a denial of all pleasure.

AC/DC—See Bisexual

Acquired Immunodeficiency Syndrome—A disease caused by one of a family of viruses which break down the body's immune system leaving it open to opportunistic infections. See HIV.

AIDS—See Acquired Immunodeficiency Syndrome.

AIDS Related Condition—A type of AIDS. A serious stage of HIV infection characterized by opportunistic infections other than those clearly associated with AIDS.

AIDS Related Virus—A strain of Human Immunodeficiency Virus (HIV).

Ambisexual—See Bisexual.

Anal Copulation—A form of sexual intercourse involving penetration of the anus by the penis. Please note that both men and women can be anally copulated. This is also called anal coitus. Slang terms include corn holing, ass fucking, Greek, and buggery.

Anal Eroticism—Finding sexual enjoyment in the stimulation of one's own or a partner's anus. See ass play.

Anilingus—A sexual behavior involving contact between the mouth and the anus. Also called anilinctus and anal-oral sex. Slang terms include rimming, rim job, reaming and ream job.

Analinctus—See Anilingus.

Anal-oral Sex—See Anilingus.

Ano-manual Intercourse—A sexual act involving placing a hand in a partner's anus. After insertion the hand is made into a fist and a thrusting motion is made. Other terms include fist fucking, FFA, and Brachio-proctic Intercourse.

Antibody—A protein produced by the body to neutralize an infection. In AIDS, these antibodies are not usually effective.

Anus—The opening at the lower end of the alimentary canal. The ring of muscles between the rectum and the outside of the body. Slang terms include asshole, butt hole, and bung hole.

ARC—See AIDS Related Conditions.

ARV—See AIDS Related Virus.

Ass—See Buttocks.

Ass Fucking—See Anal Copulation.

Asshole—See Anus.

Asceticism—See Abstinence.

Ass Play—Erotic stimulation of the anus orally, digitally, manually, with a penis or other body part or device.

B & D—Also written as B/D and BD. Short for bondage and discipline. Used by some to denote a mild form of sadomasochism, but no clear distinction exists. See also Sadomasochism.

Ball—See Coitus.

Balls—See Testicles.

Basket—Slang term for male sex organs.

Beating Off—See Masturbation.

Beating Your Meat—See Masturbation.

Beaver—See Vulva.

Behind—See Buttocks.

Belly Button—See Navel.

Benwa Balls—A sex aid consisting of small metal or plastic balls that are placed in the vagina.

Bestiality—Sexual interest and/or behavior with animals. Also called Zoophilia.

Bi—See Bisexual.

Big "O"—See Orgasm.

Bisexual—A sexual orientation where erotic and emotional

attraction to both sexes exists. Slang terms include bi, versatile, to go both ways, and AC/DC.

Blood—Liquid which flows through the veins and arteries of people. Contains various cells e.g. red blood cells, lymphocytes.

Blow Job—See Fellatio.

Blue Balls—Painful testicles resulting from prolonged sexual stimulation without ejaculation.

Bone or Boner—See Erection.

Boobs—See Breasts.

Bosom—See Breasts.

Box—See Vagina.

Brachio-proctic Intercourse—See Ano-manual Intercourse.

Breasts—Area of the chest surrounding the nipple. In women this area may be enlarged and is the source of milk production. Slang terms include boobs, bosom, tits, headlights, knockers, milkcans, teats, and mammaries.

Breeders, The—Pejorative slang term for heterosexuals.

Buggery—See Anal Copulation.

Bung Hole—See Anus.

Buns—See Buttocks.

Bush—See Pubic Hair.

Butt—See Buttocks.

Butch—Slang term to describe someone or something as masculine.

Butt Hole—See Anus.

Buttocks—The area of the body that normally makes contact with the chair when seating. An erogenous zone for some people. Slang terms include buns, rear, can, rump, nates, behind, butt, ass, duff, and fanny.

Call Girl—See Prostitute.

Can—See Buttocks.

Candidiasis—A common yeast infection which can be an opportunistic infection associated with AIDS. Sometimes called thrush when in the mouth or throat.

Celibacy—See Abstinence.

Cervix—The neck of the uterus which protudes into the vagina.

Chancre—A sore on the skin, usually associated with syphilis.

Chastity—The state of not leading an immoral life.

Chlamydia—A vaginal or urinary infection that can be sexually transmitted.

Clap—See Gonorrhea.

Climax—See Orgasm.

Clit—See Clitoris.

Clitoris—The only human organ the sole purpose of which appears to be pleasure. It is part of the vulva. Slang terms include clit, little man in the boat, and jewel in the lotus.

CMV—See Cytomegalovirus.

Cock—See Penis.

Cock Ring—A device placed around the base of the penis and testicles that aids men in getting and maintaining an erection, as well as prolonging sex.

Cocksucker—Sometimes used as a derisive term, but applies to anyone who engages in fellatio.

Co-factors—Other infections or genetic predispositions or environmental issues that increase either the likelihood of HIV infection or the progression of the disease.

Coitus—Sexual intercourse. Often used with a modifier in front to distinguish type, e.g. anal coitus, inter-femoral coitus, etc. Slang terms include fuck, hump or ball.

Come—To have an orgasm and/or ejaculation. Alternate spelling of cum. See Cum.

Condom—A sheath made of latex or sheep's intestine which fits over the penis. Used for birth control and prevention of sexually transmitted diseases. Slang terms include prophylactic, scum bag, French letter, rubber, skin, and contraceptive.

Contraceptive—Any device or procedure to avoid pregnancy. See Condom.

Copralalia—The act of talking dirty, usually in an attempt to be sexually arousing.

Coprophilia—A sexual interest in feces.

Corn Holing—See Anal Copulation.

Crabs—A form of body lice that look like tiny crabs. Usually found in the pubic hair.

Cum—See Semen.

Cunnilinctus—See Cunnilingus.

Cunnilingus—Sexual stimulation of the vulva with the tongue. Also spelled cunnilinctus. Slang terms are cunt lapping, eating pussy.

Cunt—See Vagina.

Cunt Lapping—See Cunnilingus.

Curse, The—See Menstruation.

Cytomegalovirus—An opportunistic infection associated with AIDS, but is common and usually occurs without AIDS.

D & S—Also written D/S or DS. Short for Dominance and Submission. Another term for sadomasochism. See Sadomasochism.

Detumescence—The process of losing an erection, deflation of the penis.

Diaphragm—A round, latex object inserted in the vagina to cover the cervix. Used as a contraceptive or as part of a risk reduction strategy.

Dick—See Penis.

Diddle—See Masturbation. This term is especially used to denote female masturbation.

Digital-anal Sex—Erotic stimulation of the anus with a finger or fingers.

Dildo—An artificial penis.

Dose, A—See Gonorrhea.

Douche—An internal rinsing vaginally or rectally.

Drip, The—See Gonorrhea.

Dry Kiss—Also called a social kiss. A kiss with no exchange of saliva.

Duff—See Buttocks.

Dyke—See Lesbian. Sometimes pejorative depending on context.

Dysfunction—Not functioning or failure to function. Often used to denote sexual problems.

Eat—See Oral Sex.

EBV—See Epstein-Barr Virus.

Ejaculate—The fluid emitted during ejaculation.

Ejaculation—Process of emitting semen from the penis.

ELISA—A test for HIV antibodies.

English—See Sadomasochism.

Epidemic—The uncontrolled spread of a disease.

Epstein-Barr Virus—A common virus which can be a serious opportunistic infection when associated with AIDS. Also has been hypothesized as a co-factor for AIDS.

Erection—The engorgement of the penis with blood. Can be a sign of sexual excitement. Slang terms include bone and boner.

Erogenous Zone—Any area of the body that when stimulated increases sexual excitement.

Erogeny—Pertaining to sexuality and sensuality.

Erotic—Anything that is sexually stimulating.

Estrogen—A sex hormone found in both men and women.

Exhibitionism—Sexual interest in exposing one's genitals. Slang term is flash.

Fag—See Male Homosexual. Often demeaning and insulting.

Faggot—See Male Homosexual. Also pejorative.

Fairy—See Male Homosexual. Sometimes pejorative.

Fallopian Tube—See Oviduct.

Family Jewels—See Testicles.

Fanny—See Buttocks.

Fellatio—Generally, the sexual act of stimulating a penis orally. More specifically, the penis is stationary and the mouth moves during the process. See Irrumation. Colloquially called a blow job, but the action is more sucking than blowing.

Female Homosexual—See Lesbian.

Fetish—An erotic response to an inanimate object, for example a shoe fetish. See also Partialism.

FFA—Stands for Fist Fuckers of America, not Future Farmers of America. See Ano-manual Intercourse.

Fille de Joie—Literally girl of joy or joy girl. See Prostitute.

Finger Fucking—Moving a finger in and out of the vagina, anus, or mouth in a manner similar to how a penis would be used. See also Digital-anal Intercourse.

Fist Fucking or Fisting—See Ano-manual Intercourse—This term is usually used to describe hand-anus contact, but can be used to describe hand-vagina contact. See Vaginal-manual Intercourse.

Flaccid—Non-erect, soft, especially when describing a penis.

Flagellation—The striking of a partner with an instrument, usually as part of a sexual act and usually striking the back and buttocks. The instrument is usually a whip, cat-of-nine-tails, quirt, etc.

Flash—See Exhibitionism.

Foreplay—A misnomer for any sexual activity prior to coitus.

Fornication—Coitus when unmarried.

Four-letter Word—Euphemism for any word that is generally thought of as vulgar or obscene.

French—See Oral Sex.

French Letter—See Condom.

French Kiss—See Wet Kiss.

Frigging—See Masturbation. This term especially used to denote female masturbation.

Fruit—See Male Homosexual. Used for humor or insults.

Fuck—See Coitus.

Gang Bang—See Group Sex.

Gash—Male slang term for vulva or vagina. Can be pejorative.

Gay—Polite word to refer to homosexual males or females.

Gay Men—See Male Homosexual.

Gay Related Immunodeficiency Disease—An obsolete term for AIDS.

Genitalia—Scientific inclusive term for external sex organs of either sex.

Give Head—See Oral Sex.

Glans—The head of the penis, the area covered by the foreskin in uncircumcised men.

Glory Hole—A hole in a wall or partition that a man sticks his penis through. The person on the other side then anonymously fellates, masturbates or otherwise stimulates the penis.

Go Both Ways—See bisexual.

Go Down—Slang for oral sex.

Golden Shower—See Urophilia.

Gonads—See Testicles. Also scientific term for genitals.

Gonorrhea—A sexually transmitted disease. Slang terms include clap, the drip, and a dose.

Greek—See Anal Copulation. May be used in a broader sense to include any form of anal eroticism.

GRID—See Gay Related Immunodeficient Disease. No longer used.

Group Sex—Sexual contact among more than two people simultaneously.

Hair Pie—Slang term for vulva, usually used as part of phrase "eat hair pie" referring to cunnilingus.

Hand Job—Slang term for masturbating, especially a partner.

Hard On—See Erection.

Head, Give—See Oral Sex.

Headlights—See Breasts.

Hemophilia—A genetic disease where the person's blood either does not clot or clots slowly. Only found in men.

Hepatitis—A liver infection. There are several types which used to be known as infectious or noninfectious. Now know as A, B, and non-A, non-B. All types are infectious and can be transmitted sexually by the exchange of bodily fluids. Safer Sex techniques also stop the spread of hepatitis.

Herpes—A slang term for a viral infection of herpes simplex I or II. This infection is exemplified by the eruption of painful blisters and can be sexually transmitted. There are several other viruses in the herpes family. All can be opportunistic infections of AIDS.

Het—Pejorative term in the gay subculture for heterosexual.

Heterosexual—The sexual orientation or behavior involving sex between a male and a female.

HIV—See Human Immunodeficiency Virus.

Ho—See Prostitute.

Homo—Slang derisive term for homosexual.

Homosexual, Male—See Male Homosexual.

Homosexual, Female—See Female Homosexual.

Honeypot—Slang term for vulva or vagina.

Hooker—Slang term for prostitute.

Hormone—A substance secreted by the body into the blood which controls various bodly functions. Sex hormones control menstruation, libido, and formation of secondary sex characteristics (i.e. growth of body hair).

Horny—Slang term for being desirous of sex.

Hot—Slang term for a sexual turn-on, a person or thing that evokes a strong sexual response.

HTLV-III—See Human T-cell Lymphotrophic Virus III.

Human Immunodeficiency Virus—The virus associated with AIDS which includes HTLV-III, ARV and LAV strains.

Human T-cell Lymphotrophic Virus III—A strain of HIV.

Hump—See Coitus.

Hustler—Slang term for prostitute.

Hygiene—Referring to keeping the body clean and healthy.

Hymen—A membrane that partially covers the opening of the vagina. Broken or greatly stretched after first coitus.

Immune—Capable of being exposed to a disease and not contracting it. Most immunity is temporary.

Immune System—The bodily system which fights infection by other organisms.

Immuno-globulin—A substance manufactured by the immune system to help fight infections.

Immuno-suppression—Suppression of the immune system.

Impotence—The inability to get or maintain an erection.

Infection—The state which results when a disease organism invades the body.

Infibulation—The practice of piercing the genitalia or nipples and the insertion of rings or bars ususlly for body adornment.

Inter-femoral—Between the thighs, e.g. inter-femoral intercourse or rubbing the penis between a partner's thighs.

Inter-mammary—Between the breasts, e.g. inter-mammary intercourse or rubbing the penis between a partner's breasts.

Intercourse—Euphemism for coitus, e.g. sexual intercourse.

Intra-uterine Device—A birth control device that is placed in the uterus of a woman.

Intromission—The act of placing the penis inside a partner's body, i.e. vaginal intromission, anal intromission, oral intromission.

Irrumation—Colloquially, the act of fucking a mouth. The mouth is stationary and the penis moves in and out during the act. See Fellatio.

IUD—See Intra-uterine Device.

Jacking Off—See Masturbation.

Jack Off Party—A sexual event where people masturbate either themselves or each other. Can be a safe sex technique.

Jerking Off—See Masturbation.

Jilling Off—Women's slang term for female masturbation.

Jism—See Semen.

J/O Party—See Jack Off Party.

Jockstrap—A piece of male underwear that covers the man's penis and scrotum.

John—Slang for a prostitute's customer.

Joint—See Penis. Also slang term for marijuana cigarette.

Joy Stick—See Cock.

Kaposi's Sarcoma (KS)—An opportunistic infection associated with AIDS. A rare form of cancer.

Kegels—A series of exercises to strengthen the pubococcygeal (P.C.) muscles which aid in the enjoyment of sex and ease in reaching orgasm.

Kinky—Slang term for any nonstandard sexual behavior or desire.

Kiss—Any activity which involves the juxtaposition of the lips. See Wet Kiss and Dry Kiss.

Knockers—See Breasts.

KS—See Kaposi's Sarcoma.

Labia—Scientific term for lips of the vagina, usually used to denote the genital labia minora and labia majora.

Lactation—The process of the production and excretion of milk through the nipple.

LAV—See Lymphadenopathy Associated Virus.

Lavender—A slang term usually used to denote homosexual activities or events.

Lay—Slang for coitus.

Leather—Slang for an erotic interest in leather or the sexual style of people who wear leather (i.e. S/M).

Les—Slang term for lesbian.

Lesbian—A female who sees herself predominately sexually and emotionally attracted to other females.

Lesser AIDS—See AIDS Related Condition.

Lezzie—Pejorative slang for Lesbian.

Lez—Often pejorative slang for Lesbian.

Libido—Sex drive or sexual interest.

Lips—See Labia

Load—Slang term for ejaculate, as in "shoot your load."

Love—Emotional feeling of closeness for another, sometimes used as a euphemism for coitus (e.g. making love).

Lubrication—The substance, either artificial or natural, that aids insertion of penis, dildo, or fingers into an orifice.

Lust—Desire for sex.

Lymphadenopathy—A chronic condition of swollen lymph nodes.

Lymphocytes—A cell that is in the blood and the lymph fluid which is part of the body's immune system. These cells are invaded by HIV.

Lymphadenopathy Associated Virus—A strain of human immunodeficiency virus.

Maidenhead—Polite term for hymen.

Make Love—Polite term for coitus.

Making Out—See Neck.

Male Homosexual—A man whose primary erotic and romantic interests are in other men.

Mammaries—See Breasts.

Man in the Boat—See Clitoris.

Manhole—See Vagina, also Anus.

Manual-vaginal Intercourse—See Vaginal-manual Intercourse.

Masochism—The sexual orientation where one derives sexual pleasure from receiving physical and/or psychological pain. See also Sado-masochism.

Massage—The caressing and stroking of the body for sensual enjoyment or relaxation.

Masturbation—The purposeful stimulation of one's genitals to produce sexual excitement and/or orgasm. Usually thought of as a practice done to oneself, but can be done to a partner (e.g. mutual masturbation). Additionally a person may masturbate in the presence of others, see Jack Off Party. Slang terms include beating off, beating your meat, jacking off, jerking off, jilling off, frigging, and diddle.

Menstruation—The approximately monthly shedding of the

human female's uterine lining. The menstrual cycle is the hormonal cycle that results in menstruation. Slang terms include the curse and a period.

Milk Cans—See Breasts.

Monogamy—Literally means married to one person. Colloquially used to describe any sexually exclusive relationship.

Mons Veneris—Literally means "mound of Venus." The fat pad over the pubic bone (symphysus) in the human female which is covered with pubic hair.

Mores—The beliefs of someone or group concerning the rightness or wrongness of an act or action.

Motherfucker—Slang derisive term.

Mucosa—The lining of the mouth, vagina, rectum, urethra etc.

Muff—Slang term for vulva.

Muff Diving—Slang term for cunnilingus.

Naked—See Nude.

Nates—See Buttocks.

Navel—Structure left after the umbilicus has been sloughed off after birth.

Neck, To—To kiss and hug. Also called making out.

Nipple—Structure on the breast that milk is exuded from in females, vestigal in males. Also a source of erotic enjoyment.

Nocturnal Emission—An orgasm or ejaculation during sleep. Need not be at night and can occur in women. Also called a wet dream.

Nude—Without clothes.

Nuts—See Testicles.

Nympho—See Nymphomaniac.

Nymphomaniac—A female who is supposedly sexually insatiable. Pejorative.

Obscene—A pejorative term used by individuals or groups to define depictions and/or descriptions of sexual activity which they feel is offensive. At present it is properly a legal term.

Onanism–Withdrawal during coitus to ejaculate. A misnomer for masturbation.

Opportunistic Infection—An infection that lies dormant in the body until the immune system is seriously damaged or compromised at which point the infection overwhelms the immune system and actively emerges. In conjunction with the HTLV-III (HIV) the infection becomes virulent and life-threatening.

Oral Copulation—See Oral Sex.

Oral-genital Contact—See Oral Sex.

Oral Sex—Any sexual contact between mouth and genitals. Also called oral copulation and oral-genital sex. Slang terms include French, eat, blow job and give head.

Orchis—Derived from orchid. See Testicles.

Orgasm—Sexual release following a buildup of neuromuscular tension. Slang terms include the big "O" and climax.

Orgy—See Group Sex.

Oviduct—The tube in women which conducts the egg from the ovary to the uterus.

Ovary—Female organ that produces eggs and also hormones.

Ovulation—Process in which the egg is released from the ovary.

Partialism—An erotic response to a part of the body, for example a foot partialism.

PCP—See Pneumocystitis Carinii Pneumonia.

Pecker—Slang term for penis.

Peeping Tom—Slang for voyeur.

Penis—Male sex organ which also serves the purpose of housing the tube (urethra) that conducts both semen and urine out of the body. Slang terms include cock, joy stick, joint, prick, dick, and rod.

Peno-vaginal Intercourse—Coitus. Sexual activity with the penis inside the vagina.

Period—See Menstruation.

Pessary—Old term for diaphragm.

Petting—Includes kissing, hugging, fondling, mutual masturbation, but not coitus.

Phallus—Another term for penis.

Piercing—The practice of placing various rings or bars through the body for adornment and sexual excitement.

Piss—Slang for urine.

Placebo—An inert substance that appears to have the effect of a drug. Used in tests of drug effectiveness.

Plasma—A constituent of blood.

Pneumocystis Carinii Pneumonia—An opportunistic infection related to AIDS.

Porn—See Pornography.

Pornography—Derogatory term used to describe sexually explicit material.

Pot—Slang for marijuana.

Pox—Slang for syphilis, once called great pox to differentiate it from small pox.

Prick—See Penis.

Privates—Euphemism for genitalia.

Promiscuous—An imprecise, pejorative term related to having many sexual partners.

Prophylactic—Any treatment or procedure done to avoid disease. See Condom.

Prostate—A gland that surrounds the urethra at the base of the bladder in males which, during ejaculation, discharges the greater part of the semen. An erogenous zone for many men.

Prostitute—Anyone who agrees to participate in sexual acts for money. Slang terms include call girl, fille de joie, working girl, whore, ho.

Prude—A person who is overly modest or proper.

Prurient–Literally means itching. Refers to a purportedly unhealthy interest in sexuality.

Puberty—The process where a child develops adult sexual characteristics.

Pubic Hair—Hair growth around the genitals, first appears during puberty.

Pubis—Another term for the pubic area.

Pussy—Slang for vagina.

Queen—A homosexual man who is effeminate. Can be camp humor or term of derision.

Queer—Pejorative term for homosexual.

Quickie—A sexual interaction that is of short duration.

Quiff—See Vagina.

Quim—See Vagina.

Randy—Slang term for being desirous of sex.

Rape—The coerced or forced participation in sexual acts.

Ream Job—See Analingus.

Reaming—See Analingus.

Rear—See Buttocks.

Rear Entry—Coitus where intromission takes place from behind.

Rim Job—See Analingus.

Rimming—See Analingus.

Rod—See Penis.

Rubber—See Condom.

Rubber Lovers—People with a fetish for latex of all sorts including rubber garments.

Rugae—Technical term for the folds of tissue or ridges of the vagina.

Rump—See Buttocks.

S & M—Also written S/M, SM, and S-M. Slang term for sadism and masochism, though used as slave/master also. See Sadomasochism.

Sack—See Scrotum.

Sadism—Sexual orientation or behavior where the participant obtains erotic enjoyment from inflicting physical or psychological pain on their sexual partner.

Sadomasochism—A sexual orientation and/or behavior where erotic enjoyment is obtained by giving or receiving physical or psychological pain. Slang terms include S/M, S & M, B/D, D/S and English.

Safe Sex—A system of safeguards that are designed to reduce the risk of contracting HIV or other STDs.

Saliva—The clear water-like fluid found in the mouth.

Sanitary Napkin—An object made of absorbent material used externally to soak up menstrual blood.

Sapphic—Derived from the ancient Greek poetess Sappho who lived on the island of Lesbos and wrote love poems to women. Literary term relating to lesbians.

Satyrist—Men who are supposedly sexually insatiable.

Scat—Slang term for sexual interest in feces.

Screw—Slang for coitus.

Scrotum—A pouch of skin and tissue that holds the testicles. Located just below the penis.

Scum—Slang term for ejaculate.

Scum Bag—See condom.

Semen—Male ejaculate. Slang terms include cum and jism.

Seminal Vesicles—A male gland that produces part of the ejaculate (semen).

Sensate Focus—A set of exercises adopted from sex therapy to enhance sexual enjoyment and sensuality.

Sensuality—The quality of enjoying any stroking or other stimulation which is not overtly sexual.

Seronegative—The lack of antibodies to HIV in blood, given as a result of an AIDS antibody test.

Seropositive—The presence of antibodies to HIV in blood, given as a result of an AIDS antibody test.

Seroprevalence—The number of people who are seropositive.

Serum—A component of blood.

Sex—General term for erotic activity. Also a reference to gender, i.e. the female sex.

Sex Toys—Any object used during sexual activity to enhance sensuality or sexual experience.

Sexually Transmitted Disease—Any disease that can be passed to a sexual partner during a sexual act.

Sexology—The scientific study of sex.

Shit—Slang term for feces.

Shoot, To—Slang term for ejaculation.

Simian Retrovirus—A form of AIDS found in monkeys and apes. Does not effect humans.

Sixty-nine—Slang term for mutual oral sex.

Skin—See Condom.

Slave—A slang term for a type of masochist.

Slit—Slang term for vulva. Often pejorative.

Slut—Pejorative term for a person, usually female, who has sex indiscriminately.

Snatch—Slang term for vulva.

Social Diseases—See Sexually Transmitted Diseases.

Social Kiss—See Dry Kiss.

Sodomy—Sexual acts involving oral-genital, anal-oral or anal-genital contact.

Soixante-neuf—Slang term for mutual oral sex.

Soul Kiss—See Wet Kiss.

Speculum—A device used by physicians to spread the walls of the vagina to facilitate an examination.

Sperm—The male sex cell that combines with the egg in the process of conception. A component of semen.

Sphincter—A ring-shaped muscle that surrounds a natural opening in the body and can open or close by expanding or contracting.

Spit—Slang term for saliva.

SRV—See Simian Retrovirus.

STD(s)—See Sexually Transmitted Disease(s).

Street Walker—Slang term for prostitute.

Stud—Slang term for a virile man, or one who has sex with many partners.

Swing Party—Stylized party where participants may engage

in sexual acts. Swing parties are usually heterosexual but lesbian activities regularly occur.

Swinger—Person who engages in sex at swing parties.

Syphilis—A sexually transmitted disease.

Tampon—A object made of absorbent material used in the vagina to soak up menstrual blood.

T-cells—A type of blood cell that is invaded by HIV.

Teats—See Breast.

Testicles—Sex glands found in the male which produce both sperm and testosterone. Located in the scrotum. Slang terms include balls, family jewels, gonads, nuts, and orchids.

Testosterone—The male sex hormone, found in both men and women.

Thrush—See Candidiasis.

Tits—See Breasts.

Tramp—Pejorative slang term for a woman who supposedly has many sex partners.

Transsexual—A person who believes they are really a member of the opposite sex, i.e. a woman trapped in a man's body.

Transvestite—A man who obtains erotic enjoyment from dressing in women's clothes.

Tribadism—A sexual act between two women involving rubbing their bodies together. Also used as a synonym for lesbianism.

Trichomonas—One-celled organisms that cause vaginal infections.

TS—Slang term for transsexual.

TV—Slang term for transvestite.

Tumescence—The process of getting an erection.

Turd—Slang term for feces.

Turned On—Slang for sexually excited.

Twat—Slang term for vulva or vagina.

Umbilicus—Structure that connects the fetus to the placenta.

Urethra—The tube that conducts the urine from the bladder out of the body.

Urine—A yellow excretory fluid. Unless suffering from an infection, this fluid is sterile and non-toxic.

Urolagnia—Another term for urophilia.

Urophilia—Erotic attraction to urine, being urinated upon or urinating upon the partner.

Uterus—The female organ the lining of which is excreted during the menstrual period. This is a possible site of infection.

Vaccine—A substance that causes immunity to a disease.

Vagina—A canal in females that leads from the vulva to the uterus. Slang terms include box, cunt, quiff, quim, and manhole.

Vaginal-manual Intercourse—A sexual act involving placing a portion of or the entire hand in a partner's vagina. Can include fisting.

Vas Deferens—The tube that transfers sperm from the scrotum to the seminal vesicles.

Vasectomy—The severing of the vas deferens. Used as a method to prevent conception.

VD—Venereal diseases. See Sexually Transmitted Diseases.

Venereal Diseases—See Sexually Transmitted Diseases.

Versatile—See Bisexual.

Voyeur—Someone who obtains erotic enjoyment from watching another person either naked or engaging in sexual acts.

Vulva—Female external genitalia.

Wasserman Test—A test for syphilis.

Water Sports—Any sexual act involving urine.

Western Blot—A test for the presence of the AIDS antibody in blood. Somewhat more accurate than the ELISA Test, but more expensive.

Wet Dream—See Nocturnal Emission.

Wet Kiss—A kiss in which both partners open their mouths

and stick their tongues in each other's mouth. Exchange of saliva is likely. Also called a French kiss.

Whack Off—Slang term for masturbation.

Whore—See Prostitute.

Weenie—Slang term for penis.

Wife Swapper—An older term for a swinger.

Womb—See Uterus.

Working Girl—See Prostitute.

Zoophilia—See Bestiality.

THE INSTITUTE SEX INFORMATION NETWORK
1-900-CAN HEAR

AM I NORMAL?

* Too young, too old for sex.
* Penis size; men's and women's sexual anatomy.
* Homosexuality, bisexuality.
* Sexual addition.
* What is kinky sex?
* Fantasy and pornography.

HOW TO HAVE SAFER SEX?

* Safer sex guidelines.
* Living with condoms.
* Enjoying safer sex.

SEXUAL OPTIONS?

* Deciding what you want.
* Finding and meeting partners.
* What do women want?
* What do men want?
* Negotiating for sex.

HOW TO FUNCTION?

* Ways men masturbate.
* Ways women masturbate.
* Finding time for sex.
* Anal sex.
* Oral sex.
* S/M; B/D.
* Swinging.
* Sexual enhancers.

WHAT CAN GO WRONG?

* Lack of desire.
* Painful sex.
* Coming too soon or too late.
* Erection concerns.
* Women's orgasm.
* Jealousy, anger, and boredom.

SEXUAL ABUSE?

* Child sexual abuse.
* Adults who were abused as children.

EXERCISE YOUR BASIC SEXUAL RIGHTS.
FOR ACCURATE INFORMATION CALL 1-900-CAN-HEAR
24 Hours.

A nominal charge for each call of $2.00 per minute will be added to your phone bill. Calls are handled by computer and are billed simply as 900-CAN-HEAR. No one, including the phone company, will know which messages you've listened to.

The Institute Sex Information Network
is a service of The Institute for Advanced Study of Human Sexuality and the Exodus Trust. The Institute for Advanced Study of Human Sexuality is a private, non-sectarian graduate school, established in 1976. The Exodus Trust is a non-profit California Trust that has as its sole and exclusive purpose to perform educational, scientific and literary functions relating to sexual, emotional, mental and physical health.

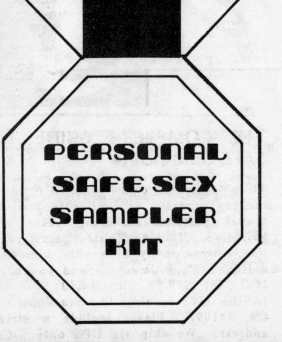

INSTITUTE FOR ADVANCED STUDY OF HUMAN SEXUALITY

THE PERSONAL SAFE SEX SAMPLER KIT

Designed to develop safer sex skills. Contains a generous collection of condoms, latex gloves, latex dams, finger cots, a chemical barrier lubricant, informational inserts and a reorder form. Send $11.95 plus $3.50 S/H to: IASHS, 1523 Franklin St., San Francisco CA 94109. Please include a street address. We ship only via UPS. CA residents please add tax.

PERSONAL SAFE SEX SAMPLER KIT

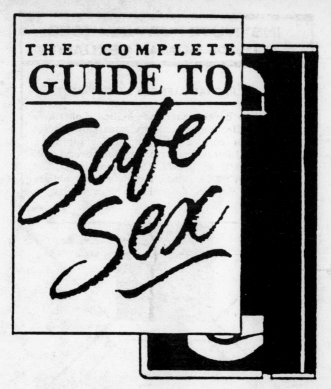

THE COMPLETE GUIDE TO SAFE SEX VIDEO

Video companion to this book. A feature-length, sexually explicit potpourri of sexual patterns following safer sex guidelines. Includes fantasy, masturbation, heterosexuality, bisexuality, homosexuality, S/M, intimacy. Send check or M.O. for $19.95 plus $4.50 S/H to: IASHS, 1523 Franklin St., San Francisco CA 94109. Please include a street address. We ship via UPS only. CA residents add tax.